Embodied Politics

Critical Issues in Health and Medicine

Edited by Rima D. Apple, University of Wisconsin–Madison and
Janet Golden, Rutgers University–Camden

Growing criticism of the U.S. healthcare system is coming from consumers, politicians, the media, activists, and healthcare professionals. Critical Issues in Health and Medicine is a collection of books that explores these contemporary dilemmas from a variety of perspectives, among them political, legal, historical, sociological, and comparative, and with attention to crucial dimensions such as race, gender, ethnicity, sexuality, and culture.

For a list of titles in the series, see the last page of the book.

Embodied Politics

Indigenous Migrant Activism, Cultural Competency, and Health Promotion in California

Rebecca J. Hester

Rutgers University Press

New Brunswick, Camden, and Newark, New Jersey, and London

Library of Congress Cataloging-in-Publication Data

Names: Hester, Rebecca J., author.
Title: Embodied politics: indigenous migrant activism, cultural competency,
  and health promotion in California / Rebecca J. Hester.
Other titles: Critical issues in health and medicine.
Description: New Brunswick: Rutgers University Press, [2022] | Series: Critical issues
  in health and medicine | Includes bibliographical references and index.
Identifiers: LCCN 2021035470 | ISBN 9780813589497 (paperback; alk. paper) |
  ISBN 9780813589503 (hardcover; alk. paper) | ISBN 9780813589510 (epub) |
  ISBN 9780813589527 (pdf) | ISBN 9780813598017 (mobi)
Subjects: MESH: Health Promotion | Transients and Migrants | Indigenous Peoples |
  Cultural Competency | California | Mexico—ethnology
Classification: LCC RA447.C2 | NLM WA 300 AC2 | DDC 362.109794—dc23
LC record available at https://lccn.loc.gov/2021035470

A British Cataloging-in-Publication record for this book is available from the British Library.

References to internet websites (URLs) were accurate at the time of writing. Neither the author
nor Rutgers University Press is responsible for URLs that may have expired or changed since
the manuscript was prepared.

♾ The paper used in this publication meets the requirements of the American National
Standard for Information Sciences—Permanence of Paper for Printed Library Materials,
ANSI Z39.48-1992.

www.rutgersuniversitypress.org

Manufactured in the United States of America

Contents

Contents

Preface

It is a bad time to question the politics of public health promotion. On the heels of a devastating pandemic that has killed millions of people worldwide, and in a country that has had the most deaths, including disproportionate numbers of racialized minorities, it seems hardly the moment to question whether we want public health experts telling us what to do and how to act. The obvious response is that we *do* want public health advice in order to keep ourselves and our loved ones safe and alive in the middle of a deadly crisis.

Yet, precisely because of the gravity of the situation and because health messages have become both ubiquitous and highly politicized, it is important to take a closer look at the politics of public health promotion, perhaps now more than ever. As many people in the United States have resisted the mask mandate and refused to social distance, compliant publics and health experts alike have questioned what is driving their behavior. Why have so many people acted contrary to the scientifically informed public health messages that are flooding the airwaves, populating the media, and being reinforced at the entrance of every shop, gym, and restaurant? At the same time, those who refuse to wear masks are calling into question the political and scientific establishments in the United States, contesting the perceived infringement on their individual liberties. Taking a step back from these debates, we can ask why those with differing opinions and approaches to health messages have clashed on social media, in political fora, and in the streets. Why do some people follow public health guidance to the letter, while others won't at all, and still others do, but only sometimes? What is it about public health promotion that, literally and figuratively, gets underneath people's skin?

As we have seen in the pandemic, health messages affirm and challenge beliefs about the individual body, society, and the body politic. They confirm and disrupt people's sense of what is right, what is good, and how they should live. These messages carry with them notions of freedom and oppression, risk and safety, responsibility and deviance, truth and falsehood. At the same time, health messages underscore questions of citizenship, national belonging, and the value and rights of a human life. For all these reasons, public health, and the messages it promotes, is about more than just science. It is also about social values. It is about teaching us how we should live—and die—together and apart.

Embodied Politics seeks to illuminate the influential force of public health promotion in our lives. Returning us to a time before the pandemic, it investigates an initiative for indigenous migrant communities in California that sought to mitigate their structural vulnerability through health workshops, messages, and social programs. Offering a snapshot in time of their programming, I reconstruct how these programs came to exist and describe how they operate. At the same time, I point out the conflicts, resistances, and counteractions that emerge through this initiative's attempts to guide the behavior and practices of indigenous Mexican migrants.

Based on two intensive years of binational ethnographic research from 2006 to 2008, *Embodied Politics* specifically focuses on the Indigenous Health Project, a program implemented by La Agencia, a nonprofit with offices in various cities throughout California.[1] Although my fieldwork ended in 2008, I continued to be involved in the organization as a board member and then as an external adviser until 2015. Since that time, I have remained in touch with many of the activists, advisers, board members, and employees involved in La Agencia's development and growth. In the years after completing my fieldwork I went to work at a medical school in Texas, where I studied how doctors are trained to deal with cultural and linguistic diversity. During that period I stopped working on this book in order to focus on teaching medical students to be ethically sensitive and culturally competent. The more I taught and interacted with medical trainees, however, the more convinced I became that the lessons I had learned in my fieldwork were relevant to their training because they troubled the commonsense approaches to bioethics and cultural competence in healthcare. The debates and controversies about public health, mask-wearing, and vaccines that occurred around the pandemic only solidified my conviction that both public health and biomedicine could learn something from my experience working with indigenous Mexican migrants.

By examining the politics of health promotion before it became such a hot button issue, I suggest that we can gain a greater understanding of health programs, practices, behaviors, debates, cultures, and controversies. While much of what is written here offers a snapshot of the time that I was in the field working closely with the organization staff, the information I provide offers lessons for today insofar as community health worker, or *promotora*, programs have grown exponentially across California and the United States, and many of the health imperatives and approaches to cultural competency outlined here remain at the core of these programs. Further, the structural racism, linguistic and cultural marginalization, and social injustices experienced by indigenous Mexican farmworkers in the early 2000s continue today. They have also had an impact on recently arrived indigenous migrants from Central America. This is to say that, while much has changed, many of the dynamics outlined in this book continue to be reproduced within and beyond the communities under study.

I write first and foremost for the activists, practitioners, philanthropists, and scholars who care about social justice, health equity, and the well-being of migrants, refugees, and indigenous peoples. But *Embodied Politics* is also for those who may not understand how the promotion of health can work against the values to which they aspire or against the values of the communities that they serve. Before I began this research, I would have found such an idea to be both scandalous and offensive. As a former nonprofit worker in a migrant farmworker community, it was clear to me that to improve their health outcomes people needed health information and health education delivered in their own language by people from their own community. I knew that the provision of this education was clearly an issue of social justice. Yet, as I came to learn, health promotion is not just educating people about their health, it is teaching them to behave, to think, and to live in certain ways—ways that are often in tension with their expressed cultural values and practices and, more importantly, that can undermine their health. This is why I conceptualize health promotion as an embodied politics.

I am also writing this book for indigenous Mexican migrants who are struggling to define and affirm their cultural values, ideas, and histories across time and space in the face of numerous, often invisible, forces that undermine both their health and their knowledge systems. I hope that this book is seen as working in solidarity with their struggle.

Embodied Politics

Chapter 1

The Paradoxical Politics of Health Promotion

In the small, gray community room behind the public library of a central coast agricultural town, a group of indigenous Mexican migrant women sit in a semi-circle on metal folding chairs. These women are Mixtec, one of seventeen ethnic groups in the Mexican state of Oaxaca. They have migrated to the central coast of California, often called the breadbasket of the country because of its agricultural bounty, for work and to seek a better life for their families. On this brisk, windy afternoon they have come to learn about diabetes prevention and to have their blood sugar level tested. Diabetes is on the rise in indigenous Oaxacan communities on both sides of the U.S.–Mexico border.[1] It is, therefore, an important health topic for this group to discuss. The health workshop is organized by La Agencia de Bienestar Indígena (The Agency for Indigenous Well-Being, hereafter La Agencia), an indigenous migrant-led nonprofit. The session is delivered in Mixtec by a community health worker, known as a *promotora*, who herself migrated from San Jose de las Flores, Oaxaca, the same village in southern Mexico as the workshop participants. Standing at the front of the semi-circle, she explains what diabetes is and describes the importance of a good diet and exercise to avoid contracting the disease.

After the promotora finishes her presentation, aided by a volunteer from the local clinic, we check everyone's blood sugar level. Donning plastic gloves, we ask everyone to line up and, one by one, we prick their fingers. We then put a spot of their blood on a white strip, insert the strip into a machine, and wait for the numbers to appear. The process is uncomfortable as neither the promotora nor I have done this before. Intentionally making someone bleed is nerve-racking. It is even more nerve-racking when they don't bleed, especially after repeated pricks. A normal blood sugar level for a nondiabetic is 140 milligrams (mg) per deciliter (dl). Blood sugar over 200 mg/dl suggests diabetes. We find that two of the fourteen women in this group have glucose levels between 140 and 200 mg/dl. We urge them to follow up at the clinic and ask everyone else to have their loved ones tested, reminding them that diabetes is a growing health concern in their community.

Once we finish the educational portion of the workshop, I ask the participants in Spanish what they have learned and how they will use the information. In exchange for allowing me to conduct research on their programs, I have agreed to give La Agencia feedback about the efficacy of their educational efforts. I also helped the promotora decide what information to include in the diabetes workshop. I am, therefore, invested in the responses to my questions. One woman answers, "In these workshops we get information and the idea that you need to know what's in your blood, how high your blood sugar is, well it stays in your head." Another woman elaborates, "Now we are thinking about what we eat and we are afraid that something is wrong with us. But once we have the [glucose] results and they say 'you're fine' we feel better." I then ask, "They say that people don't want to go to the doctor because they don't want to know what's wrong with them. Is that true?" A third woman answers, "In my case sometimes it is . . . because I don't even know how I'm doing and if I go and they tell me that I have a brain tumor and I have diabetes I'm going to get scared. In our villages we haven't dealt with this. . . . Here in the health workshops they also tell us to take care of our health because something could happen to us and it scares us and sometimes it makes our head hurt and sometimes we think 'I'm not going [to the doctor]. I'll take my medicines like I'm used to.' Because what happens if I go and I have this illness? Then what do I do?"

Indigenous Mexican Migration

In the last decade of the twentieth century the number of indigenous people in California increased by at least 25 percent.[2] This increase was not due to the high fertility rates of American Indians nor to the fact that many U.S. citizens began claiming indigenous heritage as a result of genetic testing. Rather, this remarkable demographic growth was due to an influx of indigenous groups immigrating in vast numbers from southern Mexico. Political and economic changes at the turn of the century affected migration patterns such that Mexican states with large indigenous populations that formerly had very little out-migration began seeing whole communities move to larger cities in Mexico and to the United States.[3]

The Mexican state of Oaxaca was especially affected by this trend. According to the 2000 census in Mexico, over 840,000 Oaxacans migrated to other Mexican states, and between 1995 and 2000 more than 55,000 Oaxacans migrated to the United States. The Consejo Nacional de Población (National Population Census, or CONAPO) estimated that by 2003 there were nearly 200,000 Oaxacans living in the United States.[4] By some accounts, the numbers were much higher. According to one indigenous activist, in 2006 there were 150,000 indigenous Oaxacans living in California, leading to the appellation "Oaxacalifornia," and almost half a million in the entire United States.[5] More recent estimates put the indigenous Mexican migrant population in California at about a quarter million.[6] By some accounts, there are about 1 million Oaxacan indigenous migrants in the United States.[7]

While in recent years Mexican out-migration has diminished, reaching net zero or below as a result of the combined effects of the Great Recession, increasingly strict immigration policies, and the pandemic, the years between 1980 and 2010 mark an important period when large numbers of indigenous people began leaving their communities in southern Mexico to head north.[8] The collapse of the international price of coffee, changes in the Mexican welfare system, the implementation of the North American Free Trade Agreement, the devaluation of the Mexican peso, and ever-growing cross-border social networks all contributed to this trend. These factors were largely driven by structural adjustment policies and neoliberal reforms pushed by the United States. The political and economic changes in Mexico left little place for indigenous peoples other than their joining the urban workforce in Mexico City or migrating north across the U.S.–Mexico border. As indigenous migration scholars have argued, governments in Mexico and the United States anticipated that passing the North American Free Trade Agreement would lead to significant out-migration from communities that depended on subsistence economies for their survival.[9] This is exactly what happened.

Many of those who migrated to the United States worked in the agricultural fields on the West Coast. For example, a longitudinal study by the U.S. Labor Department calculated that the indigenous farmworker population alone had grown from 35,000 in the 1990s to 165,000 by 2010. This included approximately 120,000 indigenous Mexicans working in the agricultural fields in California—about one-third of the Mexican farmworker population in the state—and another 45,000 children of these workers.[10] While an accurate population count has been difficult to come by, it is well documented that out-migration during this period led to "a 'critical mass' of indigenous Oaxacans in the United States, especially in California."[11]

Embodied Politics examines activist efforts to use public health promotion to empower this critical mass of indigenous Mexican migrants during the height of their out-migration from Oaxaca to the United States. It analyzes the political and economic values and imperatives promoted to, by, and for indigenous Oaxacans in California to ensure and insure their health as they make their way in a new and uncertain environment. It offers insights into the structural forces that undermine indigenous health and the challenges that indigenous migrants confront in getting their health needs met in the face of racism, discrimination, and stigma in the United States. At the same time, it examines the implications of using health promotion as an activist strategy to promote indigenous survival. In the face of neoliberal policies that have not only displaced them from their communities but have divested from their well-being, leaving them to take responsibility for their own health, there is much at stake in health education. Accordingly, this book seeks to understand the relief and tensions generated by health promotion programs in the lives of indigenous Mexican migrants; in La Agencia, a nonprofit that serves them; and in me as a critical and active participant.

The subjects of this book are the health professionals working for La Agencia's health promotion program, the Indigenous Health Project (IHP), as well as the indigenous migrants from the Mexican States of Oaxaca who used the health information they received to affirm and contest long-held beliefs, to debate embodied understandings, and to integrate and eschew proposed health practices. Although I am focused on the health workers and their program participants, because of my close relationship with the organization, I am very much implicated in the processes I narrate and ultimately critique in this book. Because I was able to help the promotoras in their daily work and had experience living and conducting research in Mexico, I became a (somewhat) trusted member of their team. Given this, I do not claim that I was simply a neutral observer. Rather, my presence and participation in the daily activities of the promotoras, including making phone calls to social workers, organizing conferences on indigenous culture, facilitating focus groups for La Agencia grants, researching health information, giving advice and moral support, and eventually becoming a board member, all undoubtedly changed the dynamic of what I was observing. The insights recorded in this book do not, therefore, pretend to provide an "authentic" or "objective" picture of indigenous Mexicans and their "traditions," as if such a thing were ever possible. Rather, they are thoroughly mediated by my presence and the perspectives I gained through the fieldwork I conducted in California, Oaxaca, and Mexico City.

In California I worked closely with community health workers, or promotoras, in a central coast town where I spent eight months. I also lived for six months in the Central Valley and made visits to other cities and towns with large indigenous migrant populations. I conducted twelve in-depth interviews with health workers, and numerous formal and informal interviews with local civic leaders, community organizers, clinical staff, social service providers, health practitioners, staff involved with a multimillion-dollar agricultural workers health initiative, and indigenous leaders and health promotion program participants. I conducted four focus groups with La Agencia's program participants and reviewed written materials, such as health curricula and guidebooks, that have been created or adapted for working with indigenous Mexican populations in the United States. I looked at international, national, and state policies on health promotion and promotoras, in addition to following news on health issues affecting the Mexican migrant population in the United States, and specifically farmworkers in California. Finally, I engaged in participant observation, often participating more than observing as I helped design and facilitate health education workshops, translate between Spanish and English at local clinics for the promotoras, coordinate cultural sensitivity trainings on Oaxacan cultures for health professionals, and negotiate with social service representatives on behalf of indigenous community members. As a result of my experience with and participation in the organization, I was offered and accepted a position on La Agencia's board of directors, which I held for two consecutive three-year terms.

The research I conducted in Mexico helped me gain an understanding of the health frames and references that indigenous migrants bring with them when they come to the United States, as well as to understand the politics and activism that they engage in within their communities of origin. While in Oaxaca I visited communities in and around Juxtlahuaca, Tlaxiaco, and Huajuapan de León. I conducted one focus group with thirty women in Yetla de Juárez, a rural town just outside Huajuapan de León, and five informal interviews with community health workers and doctors working in the region. I observed two health education workshops, conducted one focus group with rural promotoras, and reviewed the entire health curriculum developed by Instituto Mexicano de Seguro Social (The Mexican Institute for Social Security or IMSS) for rural populations. In addition, I conducted seven semistructured interviews with IMSS staff in Mexico City.

Some of the research in Mexico was conducted with members of a binational research team. Together, we conducted thirty-five informal interviews and five focus groups with a total of seventy-five people, many of them recipients or participants of the Oportunidades Program, a social assistance program that included conditional cash transfers to qualifying participants. Our team also observed one health education demonstration on sexually transmitted infections. I participated in a binational conference on migration and health in Puebla, Mexico. This week-long conference brought together researchers, students, politicians, health experts, and medical providers from both sides of the U.S.–Mexico border engaged in various kinds of social, political, and clinical work with migrant populations. In conjunction with this binational research, I participated in the design and implementation of a health survey for Mexican migrants living in Santa Cruz County, California.

The Paradox of Indigenous Health Promotion

The central focus of *Embodied Politics* is to reflect on the paradoxical politics that emerge within La Agencia's health promotion programs and that get worked out in, through, and on behalf of the bodies of indigenous migrants. These paradoxical politics are informed by several contradictory impulses. The first involves La Agencia's overriding mission of affirming indigenous identity, culture, and traditions while at the same time using the IHP to teach indigenous migrants to have and embrace new ways of living, behaving, and "being" in the United States. La Agencia encourages indigenous migrants to maintain and recuperate historical traditions, languages, and diets even as their health programs entreat program participants to adopt new practices and to think and behave in new ways. This first contradiction speaks to the tensions surrounding what it means to "be" indigenous within a diasporic context, or more specifically, what it means to be an indigenous migrant. It goes right to the heart of indigenous struggles to maintain indigenous traditions when many of the contextual factors that have historically provided touchpoints for indigenous peoples (ancestral lands, common lifeways, relationships with particular "scapes," and languages that emerge from those material relationships) are absent, diminished, or undermined.

The second contradiction is related to the first insofar as it relates to indigenous identities and practices across space and time. As I learned, there is no single indigenous Oaxacan culture, but rather many indigenous cultures that reflect the influences of diverse political and economic forces and imperatives interacting to shape indigenous identities, activities, and health outcomes in a particular context. Much of what it has meant to be indigenous in Mexico in the last few decades has been informed by contestations of the neoliberal policies in indigenous villages that have undermined historic land rights, devastated subsistence economies, and lacerated community cohesion through land fights and out-migration. Through social movements and community initiatives, and against a politics of *mestizaje* (the myth, perpetuated by the Mexican State, of common descent and racial harmony through miscegenation) that has tried to homogenize the Mexican nation by erasing its indigenous heritage, indigenous Mexicans have developed a strong sense of their collective identity and rights. However, in the absence of land and community solidarity to fall back on, indigenous migrants in the United States have been forced to find new ways to develop community solidarity and survive. One way to do this is through nonprofit programming like the IHP. Because of the ways funding is structured and healthy behavior is defined, however, the health programs they implement are informed by the same neoliberal values and policies that have undermined their communities in the first place. Neoliberalism thus operates as a force that both undermines and empowers indigenous communities striving to be healthy in their new context.

This leads to a third tension in their program between freedom and subjection under neoliberalism. Against the backdrop of growing anti-immigrant sentiment and the ongoing debates about health care access in the United States, health promotion has been conceptualized as one way to inform and empower disenfranchised immigrants who otherwise would not access preventive care. Defined as a behavioral social science that draws from the biological, environmental, psychological, physical, and medical sciences to promote health and prevent disease, disability, and premature death through education-driven voluntary behavior change activities, health promotion is informed by the best scientific practices in public health. Its underlying premise is that "to reach a state of complete physical, mental, and social well-being, an individual or group must be able to identify and to realize aspirations, to satisfy needs, and to change or cope with the environment." This premise is reflected in the Ottawa Charter for Health Promotion, the landmark document in the field, which defines health promotion as "the process of enabling people to increase control over, and to improve their health." Lauded as a strategy for enabling communities to take control of their bodies and behavior, the promotion of health is an important tool for supporting indigenous Mexican migrants who are often not fluent in the dominant language on either side of the border, who are largely undocumented both in Mexico and in the United States, and who live in precarious conditions in both countries.

For marginalized groups and their advocates, achieving health requires physically contesting historical and contemporary forces that have tried to erase their cultural and biological existence. Health promotion is a strategy to support this social struggle because to preserve and maintain their physical health is, consequently, to value their identities, cultures, and symbolic orders, all important identity markers that might otherwise become extinct with the deaths of their embodied practitioners. The promotion of minority health is, therefore, a way to advocate for political recognition, cultural rights, and the biological existence of marginalized groups whose lives have historically been socially devalued and culturally devastated. At stake in health promotion programs, then, are no less than the biological and cultural survival of the historically disenfranchised, the hegemony of and their resistance to neoliberal political and economic values, and the epistemic politics of public health.

Using the lens of neoliberal governmentality, critical health scholars have argued that health promotion is not as liberating or empowering as it seems, however. At least it doesn't free people up to act as they'd like in the world. Philosopher Michel Foucault defined governmentality as "the conduct of conduct," by which he meant a "way of doing things," or "art," for acting on the actions of individuals so as to shape, guide, correct, and modify the ways they conduct themselves.[12] Unlike theories that see power as a repressive force that is exercised over people, taking away their freedom and subjecting them to the will of a political actor or government, governmentality theorizes power as a productive force that operates within and around people, subtly guiding them to act in certain ways through their own desires and actions. Critical health scholars argue that health promotion programs produce certain kinds of health subjects by "conducting" their behavior and lifestyles so that they align with neoliberal political and economic values and policies. These governmental dynamics are certainly at work in immigrant communities.[13] This means that health promotion is simultaneously a way to promote social justice and freedom from oppression and a way to manage and regulate indigenous persons' behavior, thoughts, identities, and self-understandings.

I argue that the IHP is a space where these paradoxical politics emerge and are negotiated by the staff, the service providers, the philanthropists that providers interface with, and, above all, the program participants. Even as health promotion programs guide the behavior of migrant populations, I argue that these same populations exercise creativity in how they assimilate and respond to the information they receive. Like other racialized populations in the United States, the adaptive responses of indigenous Mexicans reveal a complex interplay of contestation and self-subjection when it comes to health messages.[14] Because the power dynamics of health promotion are not straightforward, it is important to highlight the strategies and techniques that indigenous groups utilize to negotiate and resist neoliberal governmentality in their everyday lives. It is also important to show how both the idea and the value of health vary based on the time and place in which health is being promoted. Understanding what health means in a particular context offers insight into how health is practiced, or not, within that context.

Unveiling the shifting values of health is part of a movement to promote the structural rather than the cultural competency of health workers and health researchers.[28] Cultural competency is broadly focused on being aware of one's cultural worldview, being open to and understanding the cultures of others, and being able to effectively communicate across the cultural differences. Structural competency, by contrast, refers to the ability of health care professionals to recognize the role that "upstream" social, political, and economic factors play in shaping the health priorities, behaviors, and outcomes of patients, populations, and systems. In other words, it pushes health care professionals to think about and understand how cultural differences, including health behaviors and practices, are shaped in the first place. Revealing the role that hegemonic political economic and social agendas play within what otherwise look like culturally competent health workshops not only adds an important and undertheorized dimension to the "social determinants" of health, but also illuminates why there may be disconnects and mismatches between the behaviors, values, and practices being promoted in health workshops and what the program participants, including the community health workers themselves, believe, expect, and practice. In other words, it helps explain why health information is not readily translated into health action despite the strong imperatives that exist to be and become healthy.

La Agencia de Bienestar Indígena

La Agencia was formed in 1993 by indigenous activists who took their firsthand knowledge of the hardships that come with crossing the U.S.–Mexico border and working in the agricultural fields of California and translated it into a nonprofit dedicated to supporting newly arriving indigenous migrants. Since its founding, La Agencia staff have spent almost thirty years developing programs that directly intervene in the social, structural, and symbolic violence that Oaxacan migrants experience throughout the migration process and once they arrive in the United States. Not only have they established a robust institutional presence in California, they have also developed strong and deep binational networks that included policymakers, academics, community organizers, service providers, philanthropists, students, volunteers, artists, and activists across Mexico and the United States. Reflecting their larger organizational mission, La Agencia's networks are predominantly focused on maintaining indigenous

cultures, increasing indigenous civic engagement, pushing back against policies in both Mexico and the United States that negatively affect indigenous
peoples, and educating the public about the unique attributes and needs of indigenous Oaxacan migrants.

When I first encountered La Agencia in 2006 they had four offices, one on
the central coast, two in Southern California, and the original office that was
established in the Central Valley. Each of these offices had been strategically
located to serve areas with large indigenous Mexican migrant populations. One
of La Agencia's primary programs, and the one I was interested in learning more
about, was the Proyecto de Salud Indígena (Indigenous Health Project, hereafter IHP), a community-based health promotion program delivered by community
health workers, or promotoras, in California, to indigenous Mexican migrants,
mostly Triquis and Mixtecs, from the State of Oaxaca.

I had contacted La Agencia because they were using health promotion as a
way to meet the everyday needs of newly arriving indigenous migrants and as
a means to affirm indigenous culture and identity against the Mexican national
politics of homogenization that sought to assimilate and appropriate indigenous
cultures as part of a mestizo melting pot.[15] For them, health promotion was a
means to gain social and political recognition for indigenous Mexicans in the
United States, and to advocate for indigenous well-being and human rights in
the hemisphere. The dual focus on biological and cultural survival at the heart
of the IHP held great political and pedagogical promise, and I wanted to know
more. How were they teaching health? In what language? What was the content
of their workshops, and how did they decide on the different themes and issues
they discussed? How were they promoting indigenous identity as part of their
health work? Did they promote traditional medicine (also called indigenous
medicine) or biomedicine? Most importantly, what were the effects of the IHP
on indigenous migrants?

In the spring of 2006 I traveled to La Agencia's main office in the Central
Valley to conduct an interview with Luz, the primary architect of the IHP.
I wanted to understand what was meant by "indigenous health" and how La
Agencia was using health as a way to support and empower Oaxacan migrants
in California. Although not indigenous herself, Luz is a Mexican migrant who
understands the challenges that indigenous Mexicans face both in Mexico and
in the United States. Because of this, she is a strong advocate for indigenous
migrants in her Central Valley community. At the time of our interview she was
pursuing a master's degree in public health and was, therefore, La Agencia's resi-
dent expert on health promotion.

Sitting behind a large desk, her petite frame dwarfed by a backdrop of books and Mexican artwork, Luz explained to me in her typical rapid-fire cadence that one of the most difficult services for indigenous Mexicans to navigate in the United States is health care. This is because when they go to the clinic or the hospital there are no interpreters who speak indigenous languages, or the interpreters that are available do not speak the appropriate dialect of their language.[16] They also have limited access to health insurance. While California allows children and income-eligible pregnant women to be treated under Medicaid, the process is complex and many people who qualify are not aware that they can enroll in this program. For those that were on a path to citizenship, they worried about jeopardizing their case by using public services and then being accused of becoming a "public charge," someone who is dependent on the support of the state rather than on their own financial resources. Because a spate of California legislation in the early 2000s required doctors to report undocumented migrants and limited migrants' access to public services, indigenous Oaxacans, like other Latin American migrants, worried about using health care services even if they qualified for them for fear of exposure to law enforcement and immigration authorities.[17] In sum, a host of social, political, cultural, and economic reasons prevented or deterred indigenous Mexican migrants from accessing health care in California.

Because the system is confusing and intimidating, Luz told me that La Agencia's promotoras spend a lot of time enrolling people in Medicaid and helping them navigate the health care system in California. They also spend a lot of time educating migrants about taking care of their own health. The health workshops they offered focused on themes as diverse as diet, diabetes, asthma, the adverse effects of pesticides, and child discipline. The workshops were both culturally and linguistically competent insofar as they were offered by indigenous promotoras who came from the same villages and spoke the languages of the program participants.

During our conversation I asked Luz what they hoped to achieve with the IHP. Her response revealed that there was more at stake in the IHP than I had at first assumed:

Rebecca: What kinds of changes can you expect to see in a community as a result of your health promotion programs?

Luz: Well, the concept of health promotion is to have the community adopt practices that get them to live a healthier life, to prevent getting sick. That's what it means to promote health. And it goes beyond going to the doctor. It has to do with lifestyles, no? So at work you take care to make sure that you are doing things right so you can prevent injuries. At home you take precautions so that there are no accidents with the kids, how you eat, you do exercise. The concept of health promotion is very wide and for that reason the challenge is to change the practices that the community has that are not very good for their health and change them into healthier practices. Lifestyle changes are the hardest because it's changing the way that you have lived—the beliefs and conceptions—including a lot of what you believe.

But we don't try to change people's beliefs. For example, if you believe in traditional medicine we don't try to say to people, "We don't [believe in it] but a lot of other people do. Traditional medicine doesn't work so you need to go to the doctor." And that's where La Agencia is different from other organizations because we tell them, "Your culture is important, your values are important, but now that you are in this country you have these other alternatives." And with the information, people make the choice, the decision, that they believe is best for their family. We don't want to change what they believe so that they forget their beliefs and they adopt something totally new. Rather we want them to complement their beliefs because this is the richness [of it].

According to Luz, health promotion is about teaching people to live a healthier life, to prevent illness and injury, to have a good diet, and to exercise. Nevertheless, as her response reveals, the IHP is promoting more than just good health, as conventionally understood. When it is targeted to a culturally, ethnically, and linguistically diverse immigrant audience, as with La Agencia's workshops, health promotion programs are also promoting behavior change that includes embracing and negotiating (1) unfamiliar beliefs, values, and conceptions; (2) diverse medical paradigms, including both "traditional" and bio (or allopathic) medicine; (3) complementary and "alternative" cultural forms; and (4) new practices of discipline and self-governance in the United States.[18]

Given La Agencia's history of activism, I had expected to hear that the changes they sought would be structural in nature, such as enrolling more people in health insurance programs and having more politically active program participants who were advocating for immigration and health policy reform. These were, in fact, important components of their program. What I did not expect to learn was that the IHP was also helping people complement and replace their traditional lifestyles, behaviors, and practices with new ones. Because one of the objectives of the IHP, and of La Agencia overall, was cultural maintenance, the emphasis on individual choice and lifestyle change surprised me.

Insofar as Luz's response emphasized the freedom of the program participants to become active health entrepreneurs who choose their health path
according to the information they receive, it generated more questions than it
answered. Did indigenous program participants actually and actively complement their cultural traditions with new health beliefs and values as Luz explained?
If so, what did this look like in practice? What were the proposed lifestyle
changes that La Agencia promoted and under what circumstances might the
program participants accept or reject these "healthy" changes? According to
which information or criteria would they make the health decisions that they
believed were "best" for their family? Finally, how could the IHP maintain and
affirm indigenous culture even as it sought to change indigenous lifestyles and
practices?

Based on my conversation with Luz there appeared to be a core tension in
La Agencia's work. They were promoting health goals that emphasize behavior
and lifestyle change, new modes of being, new forms of self-discipline, and new
individual freedoms to choose their identities and practices. At the same time,
they were promoting indigenous activist goals that emphasize the maintenance
of indigenous lifestyles, indigenous identity, indigenous practices, indigenous
autonomy, and self-determination. In other words, in their efforts to bolster
the health of newly arriving indigenous Oaxacans, the IHP was promoting a
paradoxical politics involving change and stasis, freedom from indigenous traditions and freedom to maintain indigenous lifeways, and new and old ways of
being and acting. The diverse and somewhat contradictory politics of indigenous
health being promoted in the IHP seemed to include a mix of health science and
indigenous cultural politics. How did they make sense of this combination? How
could I?

In order to further probe the paradoxical politics revealed in my conversation with Luz, I began working with La Agencia's promotoras to observe how
indigenous migrants responded to the information they received in the IHP. I also
became an active participant in shaping the content of the workshops and in
researching the health information that was delivered. The diabetes prevention
workshop described earlier illustrates important aspects of health promotion,
many of which I did not expect, that resonated with what I had heard from Luz.
First, the fact that diabetes is increasingly prevalent in indigenous Mexican
migrant communities is an outcome of the structural changes that these communities have experienced in recent years. Before Mexico opened up to free
trade and indigenous Oaxacans began leaving their communities to head north,
the word *diabetes* did not even exist in indigenous languages.[19] As a result of

free trade and the subsequent influx of new commodities into rural villages, however, indigenous diets shifted. They began eating more *comida chatarra* (junk food) and their health worsened. The same thing happened when they migrated to the United States. The accessibility of cheap, processed food coupled with their inability to buy more expensive food, including the fruits and vegetables that they picked in the fields, began to erode their traditional rural diets of vegetables, beans, and tortillas. Structural factors related to food production, trade policies like the North American Free Trade Agreement, and political alliances between the United States, Mexico, and Canada built around neoliberal economics had a negative impact on the health and well-being of indigenous Mexicans on both sides of the border. These structural changes are the reason that the diabetes prevention workshop is important for indigenous Mexicans *and* the reason that the workshop is taking place in California not Oaxaca.

Second, the diabetes workshop appears to be a culturally competent activity that is culturally affirming. It is delivered by someone from their home village who looks like them, speaks their language, and has life experiences similar to their own. Yet, as the participants' comments show, health promotion begins to erode their sense of self and identity: it changes not only how people think but also how they feel and behave. The information they receive makes them scared and worried because it "stays in your head." This mental imprint is, in some ways, the point of the workshops. Indeed, following best practices in public health, health promotion aspires to change the behavior of those it targets by making them rethink their lives, practices, and lifestyles. Thus health promotion, paradoxically, both affirms and undermines indigenous cultural practices and identities under the guise of cultural competency. It is delivered in culturally familiar ways even as it seeks to change culturally familiar behaviors. Health promotion also affirms and undermines people's health. While many of the women learned that they were symptom free for diabetes, one of the women in the group shared that just worrying about her health, as the workshop encourages her to do, gives her anxiety and makes her head hurt.

Third, health promotion is meant to empower people with the knowledge and information it offers. One of the core features of culturally competent health promotion is that it empowers people to take greater control of their health. On the surface, the diabetes prevention workshop achieves this goal. As one woman told me at the outset of the workshop, "To know everything is great. They should tell us what's good and bad about the food we eat." Before learning about diabetes and high blood sugar, the women in the group did not think about what was in their food or how their diet affected their health. They also were not fearful about receiving health information. After attending the workshop, however, the women were scared, and they only felt better once they had taken a blood glucose test and learned that they were symptom free.

Armed with the information about their blood sugar levels, they came to judge their health and well-being according to the numbers they received on the glucose monitor rather than by their own subjective sense of their bodies. That they began changing their behaviors, thinking new thoughts, and living their lives "by the numbers" at once challenges and supports the idea that the program participants were empowered by the information they received. They were empowered to act and think in new ways, but these new ways were more reductionist and economistic in terms of their self-understandings. By outsourcing their sense of well-being to a new group of somatic experts—the promotoras—the women in the group also became dependent on new forms of expertise and new, unfamiliar medical technologies in order to understand and define their bodies and their selves.[20] This dependence was exacerbated by the fact that many indigenous Mexican women have very low literacy and numeracy skills and therefore must rely on others to read and interpret the numbers for them. Given this, it is not a foregone conclusion that the health information they received or that the method of delivery through which that information was conveyed actually increased control over their bodies, made them more independent, or affirmed their cultural norms. In some senses it may have, but in others it had the opposite effect.

Finally, the exchange after the diabetes workshop demonstrates the differences between the women's experiences in Mexico and the United States. As they note, in the United States health messages targeting them are ubiquitous. They are constantly entreated on TV, by their neighbors, and through workshops like this one to pay attention to their health, to get tested, to see their doctor, and to know what, if anything, is wrong with them. As one woman explained, in their villages they haven't dealt with this. While health-promoting messages are also pervasive in the rural villages in Mexico, these messages are more often written on the sides of buildings, and they are focused on such things as boiling water before consuming it, preventing standing water that would breed mosquitoes, cleaning up garbage, and defecating in appropriate places. Unlike in the United States where health promotion is targeted to individuals based on their unique personal circumstances (i.e., "ask your doctor if this is right for you"), health messages in Oaxaca are not focused on the individual health of community members but on cleaning up an unhealthy environment, and, while these messages may cause resentments between neighbors who do and do not adhere to them, they don't incite paralyzing fear in those who receive them.

The information in the diabetes workshop may not have offered them a greater sense of control over their own bodies and life choices; in fact, it paradoxically made some of them feel disempowered and even fearful of gaining more knowledge about their health status. The participants were reticent to learn more not only because they did not want to confront the potential that they had a debilitating disease or because they couldn't readily understand the numbers and their implications but also because, without legal documents in the United States, these women would not be able to access life-saving health care or affordable treatment. Even if they could access health care through a dedicated migrant clinic, many of them would risk losing their jobs as agricultural workers if they took time off work to go to the doctor or if they revealed to their employers that they were a health liability because they had a disease that might affect their productivity or work schedule. Under the guise of being empowered by health knowledge, the women in the workshop were being reminded of how powerless they actually were given the structural impediments to healthy food, accessible health care, affordable treatment, secure employment, and legal status that they faced in the United States.

All for Health

Underlying the paradoxes of health promotion are political, economic, and social dynamics that push vulnerable migrants to embrace the health lessons they receive in order to stay healthy and productive while at the same time preventing them from utilizing the knowledge and information they gain to maintain both their health and their cultural identities. While blaming neoliberalism has become somewhat of an overused trope in academia, especially in critical public health studies, I argue that many of the paradoxes I have outlined here and the "squeeze" that indigenous migrants experience between learning how to improve their health and not being able to act on that knowledge can (and will in subsequent pages) actually be traced to neoliberal values.[21] Neoliberalism informs the global travels and translations of both health science and health philanthropy. These health forces, in turn, shape the emphasis on individual behavioral rather than structural change in the health promotion programs I studied. As Erica Kohl-Arenas has argued, this emphasis is by design. Focusing on what she calls "self-help poverty action" in California farmworker communities, Kohl-Arenas explains that philanthropic organizations will not fund radical structural change because it would go against their economic and political interests. Instead, they fund "self-help" programs, like La Agencia's health promotion programs, "that attract attention to the weaknesses and responsibilities of the poor and divert attention away from the capitalist processes that create poverty."[22] It is these same capitalist processes that allow wealthy foundation board members to become philanthropists in the first place. Even when health programs are being delivered in culturally competent ways, they are still informed by the highly economistic and individualistic approaches that neoliberalism values. Because the economic genealogy of health promotion is largely invisible, health is political in ways and for reasons that are not always obvious. For this same reason, health promotion programs may subtly work against the social justice agendas that migrant activists advocate.

Given the complex political economic genealogy of health promotion, whether or not these programs achieve their goals is an empirical question with context-dependent answers rather than a theoretical question that can be answered in the abstract. With its consistent mantras of cultural competency, behavior change, individual responsibility, and health literacy, public health seems to have emphasized theories of change over actual change while ignoring the historical shifts that have occurred within its own discipline. These shifts, in brief, have included going from advocating "health for all" to advocating "all for health." Despite repeated demands that health workers "meet people where they're at," public health has required communities to meet the desired outcomes advocated by the discipline rather demanding that the discipline advocate for the structural changes required for communities to thrive. I found this "requirement" to be true in my study of health promotion programs, even when they were delivered by, for, and to indigenous migrants.

One of the reasons that indigenous migrants embrace health promotion is because they have been historically denied access to advanced health education and comprehensive biomedical care in their rural villages. They are, therefore, eager to learn and utilize health science as a way to promote and advocate for the continued biological existence of their people. Seen as an evidence-based apolitical tool, health science was readily adopted within the IHP. Another reason they eagerly embrace health promotion is because health philanthropy has promoted it. Funding, therefore, shapes the kind of programs that indigenous organizations like La Agencia can apply for and implement. Because of the biological and financial needs of the populations they serve, indigenous promotoras echo and promote the embedded social and political values of public health to other indigenous migrants. As evidenced in the diabetes workshop, they advocate individual responsibility for health, dependence on somatic experts, quantitative measurements of success, and economistic self-understandings. Following the best practices in public health of cultural competency and social justice, they advocate these neoliberal values in indigenous languages to indigenous audiences.

Nevertheless, teaching self-responsibility for health, even in culturally competent ways, is no substitute for developing social, political, and economic structures that truly value everyone's health and that make it possible for all to access health care. Putting the responsibility on indigenous groups to change their behaviors while keeping structural inequity in place is not only wrongheaded when those groups must still live, work, and play in unhealthy environments, it is also an imposition that operates from colonial logics. For centuries, indigenous, aboriginal, and first nations people have been forced to decide between their continued cultural existence and their actual biological existence. Their purported failure to adapt or assimilate was grounds for family separation, re-education, and extermination. Because of this, indigenous peoples have been negotiating an ongoing embodied politics around biocultural assimilation, wherein they have been forced to adopt the values, norms, traditions, diets, languages, knowledge systems, and medical practices of their colonizers, for centuries. In the face of constant pressure to assimilate and abandon their own knowledges and cultural systems, indigenous people have resisted and many of their traditions and practices have survived. Although they have adapted and continued to exist in the face of significant challenges, indigenous people should not have to keep choosing between their biological and their cultural existence. One way to avoid this is for public health to adopt approaches that de-emphasize individual behavior change and to move away from narrowly conceptualized theories of health that position the individual as the central agent acting autonomously, albeit within broader social and environmental systems.

To summarize, it is both irrational and unhealthy to require that the most structurally vulnerable individuals should take responsibility for their health by changing their behaviors, altering their thought patterns, becoming more anxious and fearful, and shifting their cultural values and practices, while the structures in place—forced displacement, unhealthy diets, lack of health care access, precarious employment, undocumented status, and colonial logics—continually exacerbate their health problems, inhibit them from receiving health care, increase their anxiety, challenge their cultural beliefs, and undermine their collective sense of identity. This imperative to take greater responsibility for individual health in the face of a growing cadre of unequal and unjust structural forces is the core paradox at the heart of health promotion in indigenous communities. It is this paradox that *Embodied Politics* seeks to illuminate. Rather than spending our money and energy on blaming or changing the health behaviors and cultures of indigenous migrants, it is this paradox that activists, philanthropists, scholars, and health workers should address. Why do we think that making migrants and other vulnerable individuals responsible for their own health and well-being while creating and upholding unjust systems, exploitative structures, and colonial logics that undermine their bodies and identities leads to better health outcomes? What are the political, social, and economic rationales that make us believe such a dynamic makes sense and that convince indigenous migrants to reproduce it through their programs? How does our continual focus on indigenous culture, rather than on the cultures of health, biomedicine, or capitalism, perpetuate this dynamic?

One of my overall conclusions is that we need to collectively focus our efforts on structural change rather than on individual behavioral change. A corollary of this is that we need to rethink the cultures that we become competent about. Focusing on institutional cultures and the political economic values that inform them will teach us much more about why indigenous migrants behave the way they do than a workshop on competency in indigenous culture. Structural competency, rather than cultural competency, is what service providers, health philanthropists, and migrant activists should be learning. Until such time as meaningful and health-conferring structural changes can be achieved, however, it is important to understand and empirically document the ways that indigenous migrants negotiate the paradoxes they encounter within the health programs they participate in. How do they negotiate the competing imperatives promoted to them? What impacts do health promotion programs have on their identities, behaviors, and bodies? What would need to change so that health programs could be both culturally and biologically affirming? The answers to these questions will offer insight into the embodied politics of indigeneity in diasporic contexts and the cultural politics of health sciences.

The IHP: A Performative, Pragmatic, Colonial Contact Zone

Contrary to the idea that any one culture, including indigenous culture, determines indigenous health, *Embodied Politics* shows that there are a number of dynamic cultures interacting in every health care setting and system, including the varied cultures of the indigenous people who use that system, the institutional cultures of the systems themselves, the political economic cultures of the societies where the systems are developed and indigenous people reside, and the epistemic cultures of techno-science that inform all of these. This dynamic is captured by the idiom of coproduction, which posits that "scientific ideas and beliefs, and (often) associated technological artifacts, evolve together with the representations, identities, discourses, and institutions that give practical effect and meaning to ideas and objects." These various factors are continually emerging and mutating, coproducing each other as well as the identities, subjectivities,

and bodies of those they come into contact with through the IHP. The end result is a mixture of ideas, representations, norms, identities, and beliefs about
what it means to be indigenous, about what it means to be modern or "traditional," and about what it means to be empowered and healthy.

In order to draw out the complex and contradictory imperatives at work in
La Agencia's program, *Embodied Politics* conceptualizes the IHP as an influential "contact zone" wherein a number of competing ideas and cultural norms
come together to shape both what it means to be indigenous and what it means
to be healthy in California. A contact zone refers to the "social spaces where
cultures meet, clash, and grapple with each other, often in contexts of highly
asymmetrical relations of power, such as colonialism, slavery, or their aftermaths
as they are lived out in many parts of the world today."[23] In the context of California, xenophobic immigration policies, an inaccessible health care market,
weak labor protections, substandard housing, and social discrimination make
up the highly asymmetrical power relations that indigenous migrants face.

Attending to the IHP as a colonial contact zone allows us to see the cultural interactions that occur around health, the stabilities and dynamisms they
engender, and the identities and institutions that result. This means that the outcomes they produce have more to do with the coproduction of scientific and
social systems, historical forces, and emerging subjectivities in a context of significant structural inequity than with any purportedly essential and static char-
acteristic or culture of a particular group or people from a particular place.
Patrick Wolfe is instructive in this regard. He argues that "we cannot simply say
that settler colonialism or genocide have been targeted at particular races, since
a race cannot be taken as given. It is made in the targeting."[24] What it means to
be "Mexican," "indigenous," and "migrant" emerges and evolves within the context of the IHP.

At stake in the study of ongoing and nonlinear processes of coproduction
are new questions about what it means to live and die, to seek justice and experience harm, and to create and resist group identities in different spatial and
temporal contexts.[25] Such a theorization challenges frameworks that attribute
health outcomes to individual cultures or racial identities, like many studies of
cultural competency do, and instead elevates contextual, historical, and pro-
cessual understandings of health behaviors, beliefs, conceptions, and values.
This was apparent in the exchange I had with Luz, cited earlier.

Indeed, one of the striking things about my interview with Luz is that it
reverses commonly held beliefs about the relationship between indigenous culture and health science. We tend to think that it is indigenous culture—the
values, beliefs, practices, and lifestyles of indigenous peoples—that influences

indigenous health. Indigenous culture and indigenous exclusion from main-stream health care services are often blamed for the fact that indigenous populations have poorer health outcomes than their nonindigenous counterparts. The way to mitigate this historical inequity, many health researchers argue, is to embrace and understand indigenous culture, using it to inform the development and implementation of health services for indigenous peoples. For example, a review of sixty-two publications on indigenous health in various parts of the world found that indigenous culture was critical to ensuring community participation, indigenous self-determination, and a culturally competent workforce. The study authors explain that an intentional focus on indigenous culture in health programming, what is often referred to as "cultural competence," thus facilitates both accessible health services and indigenous empowerment.

The idea that cultural competence is central to improved health and well-being for the most marginalized groups also reflects the conventional wisdom in U.S. health care, especially when it comes to mitigating race and ethnicity-based inequities. Based on the transformational promise and curative potential of culture, cultural competence has become the gold standard when dealing with diversity issues in health care. Defined variously as a "set of attitudes, perspectives, behaviors, and policies—both individually and organizationally—that promote positive and effective interactions with diverse cultures" (Health and Human Services) or "as the ability to understand, appreciate and interact with people from cultures or belief systems different from one's own" (American Psychological Association), cultural competence has gained traction in recent decades as a way to mitigate health inequities while advancing both quality and business imperatives for health care institutions. Adopted by practitioners across the spectrum, including nurses, social workers, doctors, and psychologists, approaches that demand not only competence in but humility about, the cultural experience of patients or clients have become a defining feature of U.S. health work in the twenty-first century. The proposed outcome of this focus on culture is concisely summarized in the name of several efforts targeting indigenous and Latinx populations in California: *La cultura cura* (culture cures).

Emphasis on cultural competence is most visible in health promotion programs that employ community health workers, also called lay health workers or promotoras, to conduct outreach and education to underserved populations. Promotoras are often trusted and respected community members who come from the same racial, ethnic, and linguistic background of those they serve. They are thus presumed to be effective communicators due to their cultural competence. Because of their cultural knowledge, community health workers have been recognized by the World Health Organization and the Global Health Workforce

Alliance as an integral component of the health workforce needed for the pro-
gression of health-related Millennium Development Goals.

My interview with Luz complicates this understanding of the unidirectional
and powerful influence that indigenous culture has on health. As several decades
of scholarship across a variety of disciplines have revealed, culture is more complicated than many health studies would lead us to believe. Closely reading
Luz's comments reveals that indigenous culture is not a static "thing" that
defines and binds atavistic indigenous people to their "traditional" beliefs and
biological composition for all time. As she says, indigenous migrants have alternatives that they can and do use to complement the beliefs they bring with them
from Oaxaca. Rather than being stuck in a premodern culture, indigenous peoples
embrace and live modern lives, albeit in hybrid and heterogeneous ways.

Embodied Politics assumes such a dynamic understanding of indigenous
cultures and their health politics. One that maintains "traditional" conceptions
and values even as it incorporates and operationalizes new ideas, beliefs, and
embodied practices. This dynamic understanding of indigenous cultures resonates with scholarship that sees indigeneity as performative rather than static.
From this perspective, indigenous culture is an iterative process of doing (performativity) even as it is perceived as something that is already done (performance), taking and shedding practices in everyday life. Positing indigenous
performativity as a complex and hybrid process builds on the literature in indigenous studies that critiques homogenized notions of indigeneity and universal-
ized understandings of indigenous bodies. As Sarah Radcliffe has argued, "While
indigenous and postcolonial studies have extensively discussed liberal understandings of indigeneity's problematic, non-liberal subjectivity and about-to-die-
out corporeality, and also the resultant containment on indigenous agency, recent
literature is moving towards nuanced and situated accounts of the differenti-
ated agencies and embodiments of indigenous subjects."[26] These studies focus
on the processes of subjectivation that generate myriad ways of being indigenous in a colonial-modern context. The dynamic I seek to illuminate in this
book is the complex role that health promotion plays in shaping indigenous
performativity in California.

The idea of indigeneity as performative was reaffirmed when I asked one
of the founders of La Agencia about the tension in the IHP between a rhetorical
deployment of "indigenous culture" as a static set of traditional beliefs and values, on the one hand, and a dynamic lived process in which indigenous identity is constantly being remade in the United States, on the other. He responded
without skipping a beat, "We're pragmatic." For him, indigenous peoples will

use the cultural tools at their disposal to ensure both their biological and cultural persistence and to arrive at new truths about what it means to be indigenous. This pragmatic approach was echoed in many different conversations I had with indigenous activists. I heard repeatedly that sometimes it is strategic to essentialize indigenous culture, whereas at other times it is important to contest such essentialization in order to achieve one's political aims. The complex and ongoing entanglements and enactments of the institutional and community cultures at work in the IHP reveal that indigeneity is an embodied political process rather than a finished accomplishment. That process is profoundly shaped by, among other things, the cultural politics of health.

The New Public Health

Just as indigeneity is an ongoing process so, too, is health science, including what has been referred to as "the new public health."[27] A domain of health science that conceives of the population and the environment in their widest sense, the new public health promotes biological, psychological, social, physical, and medical health and disease prevention by focusing on behavior and lifestyle change. The primary technology for communicating this form of health science is health promotion. Within "the new public health," health has been conceptualized as "a resource for everyday life and not the objective of living."[28] As Deborah Lupton has pointed out, however, health has become both a resource for *and* the objective of living such that to achieve good health is an imperative of modern life. Embedded with this imperative are a host of familiar moral injunctions about what it means to live a good, "healthy" life. Eat right. Exercise. Don't smoke. Get more sleep. As critical health scholars have argued, the "new public health" is a sociocultural practice, a set of contingent knowledges, a moral system in ever-more-secularized Western societies and a means of establishing a set of moral tenets based on such oppositions as healthy/diseased, self/other, controlled/unruly, masculine/feminine, nature/culture, civilized/grotesque, clean/dirty, inside/outside, and rational/emotional.

Health has become a central part of the symbolic order in modern societies, operating as a sign of the Enlightenment ideals of rational control and humanistic progress.[29] The last three decades have been marked by such a significant increase in the importance of health in everyday life such that "personal responsibility for health is widely considered the sine qua non of individual autonomy and good citizenship."[30] In addition to its political effects, the "new health consciousness" serves as an "embodied replication of individual responsibility for economic well-being."[31] It thus helps people exercise their right to health while at the same time demanding that they fulfill their "duty to be well," thereby revealing that "health for all" also simultaneously means "all for health."[32]

Many public health theories attempt to explain how and why individual behavior changes and, based on that explanation, to promote individual-level interventions. In this way, public health science aligns with the neoliberal values and rationalities of high individualism and calculative reason. Some of the most well known models in this genre include the Health Belief Model, the Theory of Planned Behavior, Diffusion of Innovation Theory, the Social Cognitive Theory, the Transtheoretical Model (also known as the Stages of Change Model), the Health Action Process Approach, and Applied Behavioral Analysis, to name a few. These individual-level approaches have been referred to as "active" within the public health literature because they rely on the agency of individuals to implement social and political change. By contrast, structural changes have been referred to as "passive."[33] In recent decades there has been a growing reliance on "active" over "passive" approaches. Yet, the active/passive separation assumes that structures do not actively work on (and against) individual health. At the same time, the active/passive breakdown supports a theory of change in which individuals are encouraged to actively work on themselves, but not against the structures that harm them.[34]

Based on the best theories in public health in capitalist industrialized societies, health promotion programs promote a particular embodied orientation that includes acquiring an individual and individualist understanding of the body and self as private property to be developed, optimized, and capitalized on insofar as this embodied property is a potential site for stemming economic risk or, put differently, for maximizing social and economic potential. Within this orientation, health functions as a tool to foster the entrepreneurial capabilities of individuals so they can ensure their own well-being and financial security in a market society.

In addition to establishing an economistic understanding of the body and self, the entrepreneurial idea of health fosters particular social relations between parents and children, and between individuals in society, based on enterprise logic. It promotes a calculative attitude toward life and reproduction whereby citizens are called to take upon themselves the responsibility of managing their own well-being by continually accessing health education and health information about risk management and disease prevention.[35] This competitive *mentality* also extends to those "somatic experts," such as health care and nonprofit workers, who are in a constant battle to increase and improve their "numbers," including the number of people they serve; the revenue or grants they generate; the heart rate, blood pressure, and A1C levels of their patients and clients; and so forth.[36]

Because of this, bodies become both an ethical and a political substance: something that individuals are obligated to work on and improve as self-actualizing subjects.[37] This is what is most often referred to as empowerment. Nikolas Rose refers to this form of empowerment as "ethopolitics." As he explains, "Health, understood as an imperative, for the self and for others, to maximize the vital forces and potentialities of the living body, has become a key element in contemporary ethical regimes."[38] This health ethic "underscores approaching one's life as an enterprise," or a business, and normalizes the idea that we should all be rational, prudent, and entrepreneurial selves actively making decisions about our conduct in the perpetual pursuit of self-improvement.[39] It also underscores approaching health clients and consumers as an enterprise—an opportunity for health workers to improve their numbers. For all of these reasons, health science is neither neutral or apolitical, nor is it a static discipline.

Because of the sociopolitical power of health, Deborah Lupton encourages scholars to critically interrogate the ongoing ways that public health and health promotion contribute to the regulation of society. She writes that the covert political and symbolic dimensions of institutions promoting public health, the ways in which they valorize some groups and marginalize others, the concepts of subjectivity and rationality they privilege and exclude, the imperatives that compete with them, and the discursive processes by which they are constituted and supported should be brought to light and critically interrogated.[40] Following Lupton, this book seeks to open the black box of health promotion to critically examine its dynamic politics, practices, and implications.

As the foregoing suggests, critical research on health promotion highlights the ways that it reinforces expertise and authority in a "risk society," obligates individuals to ensure and insure their own health, and facilitates active, albeit regulated, forms of citizenship.[41] Yet, these studies tend to focus on the political rationales *at* work in health promotion programs without actually examining *how* they work in particular communities. Indeed, few studies examine the ways that health imperatives are negotiated on the ground by specific actors. *Embodied Politics* extends much of the critical scholarship on health promotion rooted in governmentality studies, which focus on the ways that health imperatives "conduct the conduct" of health subjects while neglecting to show mixed effects, resistances, and downright refusals to internalize and embody the health norms being promoted to them.[42] Illuminating these mixed responses offers insight into the ongoing dialectic between subjection and empowerment that migrants experience while also showing the localized practices of "everyday neoliberalism."[43]

In order to offer a more nuanced understanding of health promotion, *Embodied Politics* analyzes the cultural politics at work on the IHP. This analysis brings the production of racial and ethnic subjectivity, another neglected area of study in governmentality studies, to the foreground by asking what happens when the power of health science is met with the power of a hemispheric movement for indigenous autonomy in a diasporic context? How are public health imperatives, which are predominantly based on Western notions of enlightenment, positivist science, and neoliberal political economic rationales, negotiated by indigenous communities with millennial traditions and complex beliefs about the body, society, and medicine? What norms, values, logics, practices, identities, and lifestyles are proposed, defended, contested, or emergent whenever indigenous health is promoted? In sum, how are health science and indigenous society coproduced within the IHP?

Outline of the Book

A growing literature documents the social, political, and economic determinants of indigenous Mexican migrant health. Chapter 2 reviews this literature and argues that, given the hardships that indigenous migrants confront and their need to stay healthy and productive at work, La Agencia's embrace of health promotion makes good sense. The chapter describes the history of La Agencia and the development of the Indigenous Health Project as part of their larger project of indigenous cultural affirmation. It argues that La Agencia's efforts are part of a long history of indigenous resistance to structural violence that diminishes indigenous health and well-being. The embodied realities of indigenous migrants, in which they experience disproportionate morbidity and excess mortality, make health a clear choice for addressing their everyday needs and for working toward both the cultural and the biological survival of indigenous Oaxacans in a transnational context.[44] For La Agencia, promoting health is about doing social justice work.

Chapter 3 builds on chapter 2 and explains how the combination of social and economic precarity within the indigenous migrant community and the funding priorities of the philanthropic community made health promotion the program of choice. While it seems obvious that health promotion would be an appropriate response to the health inequities experienced by indigenous migrants in California, the extent to which this approach is invested in teaching migrants to take greater responsibility for their health in circumstances that are largely out of their control seems incongruous. Chapter 3 shows how the identification of health promotion with Mexican health practices made it seem both culturally and scientifically appropriate. Billed as a "Mexican" strategy for working with indigenous migrants in California, health promotion was held up as a culturally relevant intervention that philanthropists would promote and fund.

Chapter 3 outlines the travels and translations of health promotion and shows how it went from being a global project for social justice and equity in the 1970s, a project that reflects many of La Agencia's aspirations, to an individualized market-based approach in the early 2000s. The chapter illuminates the social history of the science of health promotion and shows how the meaning of health and the politics endorsed in its name have changed over time and across space from an early focus on social justice to a neoliberal focus on individual responsibility and entrepreneurship. This latter focus was the one informing health funding models at the time La Agencia was created and applying for support. As migrant bodies travel across borders, so too do knowledge systems and political strategies. Showing that health promotion can support a variety of political ideas and embodied practices invites critical reflection on its uses and implications in any given context. Just like indigenous cultures, the cultures of health are also iterative, dynamic reflections of particular times, place, and epistemes.

As chapters 2 and 3 together argue, seeking and accepting health funding come with certain constraints. Not only was the focus on health a necessary strategy for mitigating the structural violence that migrants face, but La Agencia's focus on health occurred at the same time as the rise in "self-help poverty action" supported by health philanthropists in response to a shrinking welfare state and rising health care costs in the United States. By developing health programming, La Agencia's architects were able to capitalize on the newly available health funding while advancing both their advocacy and their community work. Nevertheless, support for health programming was increasingly targeted toward specific diseases, and nonprofits were expected to fulfill the agendas of their funders or jeopardize further support. As a result, grassroots indigenous organizations were not able to design or implement the programs they desired, especially if it meant challenging powerful economic actors like the billion dollar agricultural industry. Further, the prohibition on lobbying and political advocacy by U.S.-based nonprofits meant that La Agencia's leadership was wary of ever appearing too political in their programs and thus avoided any appearance of political advocacy. This concern sometimes put their activities at odds with their partner institution, an indigenous social movement organization, as the latter advocated for political and economic reforms while the former tried to avoid upsetting powerful political and economic actors by adhering to the status quo.

These two chapters trace the different logics or political *mentalities* that converge to shape La Agencia's Indigenous Health Project. They also reflect a reversal of the commonly held belief that health follows identity. Instead of treating indigenous knowledges and cultures as instances of quaint folk theory held by members of a primitive culture, as much Western health scholarship on cultural competency does, the analysis makes Western structures and systems of knowledge the object of critique and inquiry.[45] Focusing on the structures and systems that inform our notions of health reveals the forces that indigenous migrants must negotiate within and on behalf of their bodies and identities. On the one hand, we see a significant need for health interventions that will mitigate the structural violence and vulnerability that indigenous migrants experience. Within this context, health is a culturally relevant social justice project that promotes the flourishing of indigenous populations. On the other hand, however, we see that the health-promoting strategy being used to mitigate the effects of a brutal neoliberal political economy that has caused significant out-migration and structural vulnerability for indigenous Oaxacans is itself promoting neoliberal forms of politics, citizenship, and subjectivity. It is promoting these things in indigenous languages by indigenous health workers. Taken together, chapters 2 and 3 offer us an opportunity to identify the paradoxical politics at the heart of the IHP and to reflect critically on the epistemological, political, social, economic, and cultural underpinnings of health promotion as a means to deal with indigenous suffering and to promote indigenous identity.

Chapters 4, 5, and 6 offer a more fine grained analysis of the everyday ways that La Agencia's program participants, staff, and affiliated community members negotiate the politics of health promotion. Beginning with a top-down perspective that looks at how La Agencia's programs are shaped by health funders, chapter 4 employs the idea of audit culture to argue that accounting and management strategies inform how health workers understand themselves and their program participants, or "clients." A quintessential marker of neoliberal imperatives, funder demands for accountability shift the program's focus from more relational and qualitative aspects of health, characteristics desired by La Agencia staff and program participants, to what one employee described as a focus on "numbers, numbers, numbers." Not only are ideas about the efficiency, productivity, and success of health workers at stake within this organizational audit culture, but, as the chapter shows, this mandate also generates competition between health workers of different ethnicities for resources and participant numbers. The focus on numbers and written documentation also corresponds to a concern with accountability and transparency from within the indigenous leadership, however. Because of past lessons learned about corruption and fraud, indigenous movement leaders argued that they need to be accountable to their base and transparent to each other. Chapter 4 shows how neoliberal audit culture, health cultures, and indigenous identities are mutually entangled, productive, iterative, and reinforcing.

Chapter 5 examines a core policy strategy for addressing racial and ethnic inequities in health in the United States. Cultural competency has been embraced by health institutions and health providers as a means to attend to the unique cultural, linguistic, and literacy needs of diverse populations. Through the Indigenous Health Project, La Agencia has been a trendsetter insofar as the organization has taken responsibility for educating health providers about the ethnolinguistic diversity of indigenous Oaxacans and about the challenges they face living in the United States. This chapter analyzes La Agencia's efforts to make health providers more conscious of their cultural biases. Illuminating the tensions at work in cultural competency, the chapter argues that La Agencia's efforts to promote indigenous culture as a way to protect indigenous health are hindered by their inability to openly discuss the power iniquities that shape indigenous health outcomes. Rather than talking about racism, xenophobia, or the history of colonization, as they would like, La Agencia staff focus on less overtly political topics, such as language differences and ethnic dress. They do this for fear of losing the funding and support of their interlocutors should their presentation be perceived as too politically charged. The same neoliberal imperatives that make them reliant on competitive funding and responsive to the quantitative measures of success demanded by their funders keep them from offering a more nuanced account of why they need that funding in the first place. This means that even as the programs are touted as culturally and linguistically competent because they are delivered by indigenous health workers, the values, beliefs, and practices promoted in these programs are as much shaped by the cultural norms of their audience and the economic imperatives of their organization as by indigenous cultural orientations and worldviews.

Chapter 6 returns us to the overall objectives of the book and describes some of the ways that La Agencia has evolved its thinking and practices as time has gone on. This concluding chapter argues that, despite the advances made by both La Agencia and its sister organization, there remains much work for all to do in order to ensure and insure the health of indigenous Mexican migrants.

Chapter 2

Structural Violence, Migrant Activism, and Indigenous Health

> We are not people who were "discovered"
> by the Spaniards, the Americans or anyone
> else. . . . We are people in struggle!

Structural Violence

A lot of sad things happened at the border. People were assaulted and women were raped by coyotes. People were deported and had no money. They had to ask for money. Fleeing the border patrol was the most vulnerable experience I faced, then paying the smuggler two thousand dollars and having to work like a slave to pay the debt. I was thinking that crossing the border my life was going to improve, and then my heart broke and I started crying, as I am now. This new place was totally different. I spent my first horrible winter here in extreme cold. I had to get up early, go outside, and work in that cold. I worked about nine to twelve hours a day. I had to pay my bills and save money to pay my debt to the smugglers.

Because of the hard work and the weather, I didn't want to stay here. I was depressed and cried, but who was going to pay my debt? I had to resign myself to the idea that I wouldn't be able to go visit my family, my village. I had to travel to Washington State where I worked in the rain all day. Sometimes they gave us big trash bags so we wouldn't get wet, but it didn't help at all. We made jokes because we didn't want to feel bad. Being a woman working in the field is harder than being a man because we do two jobs. We do all the work at home and take care of the children before and after work. Before learning my rights, I met a labor contractor that humiliated us, including me. Once a foreman told me that he couldn't pay me what he paid the men because, as a woman, I didn't have the same strength as a man, and he told me I couldn't do anything about it because I was undocumented in this country.

Perla, a Mixtec woman from the village of San Miguel Cuevas, Oaxaca, Mexico, gave this account about crossing the border and then living and working in the United States. During a public presentation about indigenous farmworker women, she began by explaining that approximately 80 percent of her village now resides in the United States. Her experience at the border, as a woman, as a farmworker, and as an undocumented indigenous migrant in the United States is not unique. Estimates of the number of indigenous Mexican migrants vary. In 2007, researchers guessed that there were between 350,000 and 400,000 migrants from Oaxaca in California, 80 percent of whom were indigenous.[1] In 2010, the *Los Angeles Times* reported that there were approximately 300,000 Zapotecs in Los Angeles County alone.[2] By some accounts there are over 1 million Oaxaqueños living throughout the United States.[3] These numbers mean that, over the last few decades, hundreds of thousands of indigenous Mexican migrants have experienced the depression, the sense of rightlessness and enslavement, the racism and sexism, the economic exploitation, the harsh working conditions, and the terrifying border experiences Perla described. And, as she explained, women withstand the worst of these violent and humiliating assaults.

As Perla's experience illustrates, racial inequity, chronic poverty, food insecurity, harsh labor conditions, economic exploitation, violence, and unequal gender relations are all part of the migration experience and so, therefore, is the social, physical, and emotional suffering that comes with these circumstances.[4] Physician and anthropologist Paul Farmer refers to this host of offensives against human dignity and human rights as "structural violence."[5] He explains that structural violence includes extreme and relative poverty, social inequalities ranging from racism to gender inequality, and the more spectacular forms of violence that are uncontestedly human rights abuses.[6] For Farmer, human rights violations, including violations of social and economic rights, as well as civil and political ones, are not accidents nor are they random in distribution or effect. He explains, "Rights violations are, rather, symptoms of deeper pathologies of power and are linked intimately to social conditions that so often determine who will suffer abuse and who will be shielded from harm."[7]

The social and economic conditions that indigenous migrants experience interact in complex ways with their bodies such that situations of chronic stress can negatively affect both their endocrine and their neural systems, actually inducing sickness. The term "allostatic load" describes the negative feedback loop between contextual and biological factors that chronic stress engenders, leading to cumulative physiological degradation and the acceleration of disease processes.[8] Clarence Gravlee describes this feedback loop as the way that race *becomes* biology.[9] Pushing back against the idea that genetics is the primary determinant of health, Gravlee argues that social inequalities shape the biology of racialized groups. Nancy Krieger uses the term "embodiment" to describe the ways that living organisms, including humans, literally incorporate their worlds biologically. She explains, "From population patterns of health, disease, and wellbeing it is possible to discern the contours and distribution of power, property, and technology within and across nations, over time."[10] Their work shows how pathologies of power become embodied pathologies. Considering this, the indigenous fight against structural violence is literally to *lucharle por la vida* (to fight for one's life), as migrants from the Oaxacan town of San Miguel Tlacotepec have explained.[11]

Indigenous migrants do all that they can to take care of themselves and their families despite the forces that undermine their health. Indeed, the long hours of hard work and the precarious and injurious border crossings that they endure attest to their fortitude, as do the creative strategies they deploy to deal with their circumstances. Wearing a garbage bag in the rain and using humor to lighten the mood are some of the everyday ways that indigenous migrants contest their inequitable conditions and find the strength to continue working and living in the United States when they would rather return home. These more personalized resistance strategies are not the only ones they use, however. As Perla explained, she was humiliated "before learning her rights." Her situation improved when she learned about her human and labor rights from a farmworker advocate working with California Rural Legal Association, a legal advocacy organization in California. Once she became politically conscious, Perla began to contest both the individual mistreatment she received in the fields and the structural inequities that she and her coworkers experienced. She even became an advocate herself, teaching other farmworker women about their rights and giving public talks on the migrant experience.

This chapter describes the structural violence that indigenous Mexicans experience both in Mexico and once they arrive in the United States. It links this violence to health outcomes, offering context for why indigenous migrants embraced health as the way to respond to the assaults on their dignity and human rights and as a means to fight for social justice. As more than four decades of scholarship on indigenous Mexican out-migration have shown, multiple social, political, and economic forces combine to produce the embodied vulnerability that indigenous Oaxacans suffer. As this research also illustrates, the precarity, suffering, and death that result were anticipated outcomes of neoliberal policies adopted both in Mexico and in the United States.

In addition to showing how indigenous migrants are rendered vulnerable to the vicissitudes of a pernicious neoliberal political economy and the violence of historic racism, this chapter also highlights their responses to that vulnerability. Not powerless victims, indigenous peoples have always sought strategies to protect themselves against violence and oppression and to promote their health and flourishing. By detailing how La Agencia grew out of an ethnicity-based indigenous social movement, the second half of this chapter highlights indigenous strength, resistance, creativity, and survival in the face of structural violence. If the effects of this violence are manifested in the bodies of indigenous migrants, then the first line of defense for migrant activists is to protect those bodies. It makes sense, then, that indigenous migrants would focus on health as a way to fight for their lives. The Indigenous Health Project (IHP) is one way to do that.

Pathologies of Power: Trade Policies

Indigenous Oaxacans began leaving their communities in the 1940s to work in the agricultural fields of the neighboring state of Veracruz. By the 1960s they had begun working their way north to Morelos and then on to Mexico State, Sonora, Sinaloa, and Baja California. In each of these states they primarily worked in agriculture. During this twenty-year period, small groups of Oaxacans had also migrated to the United States through the Bracero Program. The number of cross-border indigenous migrants increased in the 1970s.[12] The Mexican economic crisis in the 1980s, the 1986 Immigration Reform and Control Act, the effects of the Mexican peso crisis in 1994, and especially the North American Free Trade Agreement (NAFTA), put into effect in January of that same year, turned what had been a slow trickle into a "critical mass" of indigenous migrants in the United States.[13]

The lowering of trade barriers associated with NAFTA devastated the agricultural economy for indigenous farmers who could no longer grow corn or other subsistence crops more cheaply than they could buy imported products from subsidized U.S. farmers.[14] Journalist David Bacon describes the effects on rural Mexicans:

> Corn imports rose from two million tons to more than ten million tons from 1992 to 2008. NAFTA prohibited price supports, without which hundreds of thousands of small farmers found it impossible to sell their corn or other farm products for what it cost to produce them. Mexico

imported 30,000 tons of pork in 1995, and by 2010 that had grown to
811,000 tons, costing 120,000 jobs. The World Bank in 2005 found that
the extreme rural poverty rate of 35 percent in 1992–94, prior to NAFTA
taking effect, jumped to 55 percent in 1996–98, after NAFTA was in place.
By 2010, 53 million Mexicans were living in poverty, about 20 percent
in extreme poverty, almost all in rural areas.[15]

Because Mexico's asymmetrical integration into the North American economy
through NAFTA had a detrimental impact on its agricultural self-sufficiency and
labor sovereignty, it led to significant increases in out-migration.[16] Ximena Avell-
aneda Díaz, president of the women's studies group "Rosario Castellanos,"
located in Oaxaca City, described the effects: "Close to starvation, many peasants were forced off the land, only to augment the pool of unemployed already
in overcrowded cities, where the so-called informal economy grew by leaps and
bounds."[17] Many of those who were forced off their land pushed farther north
to Baja California, eventually ending up in a diverse number of U.S. states, including California, Oregon, Washington, Alaska, Nevada, Texas, Florida, Illinois,
and New York.[18] The *San Jose Mercury* describes their trajectory in the United
States and the effects on their communities back home: "Hispanic Indians often
follow berry crops from Ventura County north to the Willamette Valley in Oregon.
They work in restaurants and the garment industry in Los Angeles. They travel
to the Carolinas to work in chicken-processing plants, and to New York City,
where they work in the hotel industry. This diaspora is emptying villages in
the Mexican states of Oaxaca, Chiapas, and Guerrero."[19] Jonathon Fox and Gaspar Rivera Salgado explain that this forced displacement was anticipated by the
Mexican government, "Since implementation of the North American Free
Trade Agreement (NAFTA), the government's rural development strategy has
been based on the assumption that a large proportion of the rural poor would
move either to the cities or to the United States."[20] Indeed, for indigenous Mexicans, migration was an "escape valve" from the high levels of poverty and marginalization in regions where their land could no longer guarantee food and
sustenance.[21] Though the trade agreement emphasized free exchange across the
border, rural Mexican farmers were no longer able to compete with products
coming from the United States. Not only did NAFTA lead to the displacement
of thousands of people, it failed to promote the economic growth and wide-
spread employment in Mexico that were promised. Instead, the benefits of the
three-country trade deal accrued mostly to private U.S. firms, signaling both the
regulated and uneven nature of "free" trade for the Mexican state.[22] While goods
and money could freely cross borders under NAFTA, bodies could not. People

often had to pay human smugglers thousands of dollars to help them get to the United States, and they had to undertake a journey that could cost them their health and their lives. As the rural indigenous population learned, free trade is not free.

Dying to Survive: Border Policies

Out-migration was one of the primary strategies used by indigenous communities in the 1990s and early 2000s to resist the effects of structural violence caused by a neoliberal political economy that was encroaching on their villages. Availing themselves of this strategy, however, opened them up to more violence at the border and in the United States. Because out-migration of peasant farmers was a foreseen effect of free trade, NAFTA was accompanied by reinforcement of the U.S.–Mexico border. Months after NAFTA was passed, U.S. president Bill Clinton signed into law Operation Gatekeeper, a strategy that sought to prevent Mexican immigration through deterrence by militarizing the border in and around San Diego, California. According to Joseph Nevins, Operation Gatekeeper "was the administration's answer to the massive disruption in Mexico's rural and small business sectors brought about by growing economic liberalization, a process greatly intensified by the North American Free Trade Agreement."[23] In light of the anticipated disruptions, the Immigration and Naturalization Service (now the U.S. Citizenship and Immigration Services) commissioner, Doris Meissner, argued to Congress in November 1993 that responding to the likely short- to medium-term impacts of NAFTA "will require strengthening our enforcement efforts along the border, both at and between ports of entry."[24]

In the hopes that unauthorized migrants would be deterred from coming to the United States, the number of border control agents was increased, surveillance measures were added, and border walls were constructed. Effectively "weaponizing" the desert, Operation Gatekeeper forced cross-border migrants to traverse dangerous desert terrain under extreme conditions. Rather than deterring people, then, the overall outcome of this policy was more migrant deaths. Calling Operation Gatekeeper a death trap, Bill Ong Hing, a professor of law at the University of California, San Francisco, explains the effects of this approach: "The number of entries and apprehensions did not decrease, and the number of deaths due to dehydration and sunstroke in the summer or freezing in the winter surged dramatically. Whereas in 1994, fewer than 30 migrants died along the border; by 1998, the number had risen to 147; in 2001, 387 deaths were counted; and in 2012, 477 bodies were found. From 2007 to 2013, over 2,000 known migrant deaths occurred along the Mexico–Arizona border."[25] The International Organization for Migration puts border deaths at 398 in 2016, 412 in 2017, and

283 in 2018.[26] In 2020, the remains of 227 people were found in Arizona alone, the deadliest year to date for the migrant deaths in that state.[27] These estimates are likely low, however, since they reflect only the deaths that the border patrol deals with directly and not those occurring on the Mexican side of the border. They also do not account for those people whose bodies are never recovered. While the number of border crossings in recent years has drastically diminished, the high number of border deaths has persisted because of the deterrent measures put into place by the United States.[28] The overall effect of decades of prevention through deterrence policies, as the Mixtec community leader in Greenfield, California, so aptly explained to me, is that "migrants are dying to survive because many of them die at the border."

Territorial Sovereignty and the Right to Self-Determination: Land Policies

The fact that the escape valve for forcibly displaced populations is actually a death trap is part and parcel of structural violence. As Farmer explains, the more spectacular human rights abuses against vulnerable populations, like those that result from a fortified border, are often punishment for their efforts to escape structural violence.[29] In addition to looking for work, many indigenous migrants came to the United States in order to escape violence at home, where the economic and political dynamics had increased territorial disputes and bred civil war. In 1991 the Salinas government in Mexico "passed a reform law that both permitted and encouraged privatization of the *ejido* lands, opening them up to foreign ownership."[30] The ejido system, put in place through Mexico's 1917 Constitution, guaranteed the collective ownership and use of lands for indigenous groups. "Since the *ejido* provided the basis of collective security among indigenous groups, the government was, in effect, divesting itself of its responsibilities to maintain that security."[31] This divestment and increased privatization of common land led to infighting within and between indigenous communities that continues today. Indeed, in 2019 the mayor of Tlaxiaco, Oaxaca, Alejandro Aparicio Santiago, was shot on the way to his first official meeting at city hall. The cited reason for the shooting was land disputes.[32]

As many of those I interviewed for this book explained to me, their communities of origin have experienced high levels of violence and repression in the last few decades. Murder and gun violence have directly impacted the lives of those involved with the IHP. For example, the fathers of two community health workers (*promotoras*) I worked with closely during my field research, one Triqui and the other Mixtec, were killed. The Triqui woman's father was killed during the time I was doing research. He was shot while sitting in front of his home in the small village of Río Venado, Oaxaca, talking with his landlady. There was no known cause for the murder. He had just returned to Oaxaca from California two weeks prior to his death. The Mixtec man, a large landholder, was killed years earlier. His daughter reported that the cause of his death was *celos* (jealousy) over his wealth. In a third example, a Mexican professor with whom I was traveling in Oaxaca for research reported that her colleague, a Mexican political scientist who had been working in Oaxaca, had been detained, sent to another state, and tortured. Part of the torture included cutting off several of her fingers.

The violence and abuse in Oaxaca stems from centuries of racism from those organizations and actors that have defined indigenous culture as harmful and have painted indigenous groups as savages incapable of self-rule. As a result of this historic racism, indigenous Mexicans face discrimination and oppression in their daily lives no matter which side of the border they live on. Vivian Newdick explains, "In the United States, in Mexico, in Afghanistan, examples abound of discourses of blaming culture for bad behavior."[33] The idea that indigenous culture is a drag on both democracy and development has led to the idea that indigenous ways of living should undergo radical reform.[34] These discourses too often conflate the effects of poverty and inequality with cultural difference while masking the violence that has led to such differences. Farmer elaborates on this point, writing that "The abuse of the concept of cultural specificity is particularly insidious in discussions of suffering in general and of human rights abuses specifically: cultural difference, verging on a cultural determinism, is one of several forms of essentialism used to explain away assaults on dignity and suffering."[35]

Racism and social exclusion played a strong role in the violence that led to significant Triqui out-migration. Unlike their Mixtec counterparts, the Triquis of Oaxaca did not start migrating until the violence in their communities became too much to bear. Under the thumb of local political bosses and ignored by the federal government, they had little agency in the political decisions affecting their communities. This led to a struggle for autonomy that ended up in a bloody war. Caught in a context of political submission, territorial disintegration, economic exploitation, racial discrimination, and social exclusion, they began to fight with each other and against the local political bosses.[36] David Bacon has written that although violence in the Triqui region was escalating, the federal government refused to intervene. He cites indigenous scholar, Gaspar Rivera-Salgado, as attributing the problem to the dual problem of racism and lawlessness. "The violence is created by a lack of the assertion of the rule of law. But the government has excused its failure to stop it with such racist ideas as 'Triquis are savages and uncivilized.'"[37] Many of those who left their communities went to Oaxaca City and joined a burgeoning teacher's strike. Rather than respond to their collective demands for educational support and security in their communities, however, the government responded to the strike with weapons and teargas. The insecurity at home and the violence in Oaxaca City drove many Triquis north to Baja California and then across the U.S.–Mexico border.

In the last few decades, drug gangs have moved in to battle over territory and drug smuggling routes in Oaxaca, making it unsafe to live there for the few Triquis that remain and undesirable for those who have migrated to return home.[38] Life for those who left is not much better, however. The drug violence, a lack of decent education, economic exploitation, and the impunity enjoyed by local political leaders have plagued the Triqui in Baja California, the largest Triqui community outside Oaxaca. "In such grim surroundings, many of the community's older generation long to return to Oaxaca and have petitioned both the federal and state governments to address the violence that keeps them from their cultural homeland," to no avail.[39]

The violence in Oaxaca has especially affected indigenous women. For example, in the early 2000s, Oaxaca was one of the top five entities with the most violence against women in Mexico and number one for women who experience violence in their childhood."[40] More recently, there has been a marked rise of femicide in Oaxaca disproportionately affecting indigenous women.[41] This violence follows them throughout their migration trajectory, where they confront gender subordination from within the indigenous community and from the larger society. The militarization of the U.S.–Mexico border perpetuates this violence.[42] As Sylvanna Falcón has documented, women are routinely and systematically subjected to rape as a result of border militarization.[43] This strategy is informed by the military doctrine of low-intensity conflict.[44] "Constructed by the U.S. military-security establishment to target Third World uprisings and revolutions, particularly in Central America, LIC [low-intensity conflict] doctrine advocates unconventional, multifaceted, and relatively subtle forms of militarization and emphasizes controlling targeted civilian populations."[45]

One of these unconventional control strategies is the sexual domination of women's bodies. As Falcón explains, "In the case of rapes at the U.S.–Mexico border, migrant women's bodies denote an 'alien' presence subject to colonial domination by U.S. officials. Their bodies represent a country over which the United States has maintained long-term colonial rule resulting in a symbolic connection between women's bodies and territory."[46] Women migrants are also raped by the traffickers that smuggle them across the border. So prevalent is the incidence of rape that many women start taking birth control before they begin their northward migration, knowing that they will likely be raped before their journey is through. This "double tax," in which women pay money to be smuggled across the border and then pay with their bodies to ensure that they make it, has become a routinized part of the political economy of migration.[47]

Ineligible for Personhood: Citizenship Policies

As the foregoing illustrates, shifts in trade, land, and border policies have negatively affected the lives of indigenous Mexicans, causing them to experience high levels of violence and abuse, as well as a continuous denial of their rights. Fox and Rivera-Salgado explain, "*Both* in the United States *and* in Mexico, indigenous migrants are subordinated *both* as migrants *and* as indigenous people, economically, socially and politically." As a result, they "are excluded from citizenship rights in either country."[48] In Mexico, this denial of citizenship is manifest in government neglect of basic infrastructure in rural communities, including access to clean drinking water, sewage systems, garbage removal, and health services; in the outright oppression of indigenous movements struggling for social justice and government accountability; in the forced displacement of entire indigenous communities as a result of NAFTA and land reform; and in sterilization campaigns that target poor indigenous women.[49]

The denial of citizenship rights for migrants in the United States is linked to historic shifts in the way migrants have been framed. Under the Bracero Program migrants were considered laborers and were regulated as such. When immigration fell under the jurisdiction of the Department of Justice, undocumented migrants were framed as criminals. After the events of 9/11, immigration came under the Department of Homeland Security. As a result of this change, migrants were framed both as illegal criminals and as potential terrorists. Undocumented immigrants and terrorists have since been conflated in the dominant discourse despite many of the people involved in 9/11 having received permission to be in the United States and none being of Latin American origin. The idea that Mexican migrants are laborers who were initially invited under the Bracero Program by the United States to do necessary work that bolstered the nation in a time of war, and who continue to bolster the nation by doing low-wage work and paying taxes into a system that returns few social or political benefits to them, has been obscured from mainstream discourse. Instead, by migrating in search of economic and social stability, indigenous Mexicans become the targets of policies and practices that punish them for their poverty, legal status, cultural identities, and, as Farmer's theorization illuminates, their attempts to escape situations of structural vulnerability. Such legalized discrimination is possible because in the United States Mexican migrants are dehumanized by legal and political frameworks that continually frame them as criminals, illegals, and sexual predators.⁵⁰

Lisa Marie Cacho argues that poor people of color are affected most often and most intensely when criminal and immigration policies are altered to be more efficient but less humane.⁵¹ This happens because undocumented immigrants, and other "criminal" groups, are treated as obviously and intentionally breaking the law. They are framed as criminals, people who break the law because of a character flaw or some inherent proclivity for trouble, rather than as people whose identity is an *effect* of the law or is produced by the law. That is, although the criminalization of migrants is an effect of changing legal structures and anti-immigrant discourses, the identity of "criminal" or "illegal" is seen as inherent to the person or population and not as an outcome of the system. Framed as "illegal criminals" because they lack legal authorization to be in the United States, undocumented migrants become "ineligible for personhood" once they cross the border.

Being "ineligible for personhood" means living in a liminal state of rightlessness in which a population is subjected to laws but is refused the legal means to contest those laws and denied both the political legitimacy and moral credibility necessary to question them.⁵² Not only that, but because they are already defined as criminal and illegal, they are subject to increased suspicion, scrutiny, and intervention. Anthropologist Lynn Stephen elaborates this situation for Oaxacans: "Undocumented workers and others who are read as undocumented in the United States and increasingly as supposed possible terrorists have been living in a world of surveillance and limited personal liberties for quite some time. They live in a contradictory state of trying to maintain invisibility while simultaneously being the object of significant surveillance at different points in their journey and work experiences."⁵³

In a climate characterized largely by anti-immigrant sentiment, indigenous migrants attempt to remain invisible so as to avoid deportation. This takes a toll on their mental health. As a doctor in Oaxaca noted, "Because things are calmer here, it's easy to notice how a returned migrant has been changed by his experience over there. It takes them two to three months to lose the sense that they are being followed, to lose the nervousness."⁵⁴ At the same time, their injurious life circumstances are made invisible by social structures that naturalize their position at the bottom of social, economic, health, and labor hierarchies.⁵⁵

Anti-immigrant discourses and the denial of citizenship rights in the United States make it so that even when indigenous Mexicans take responsibility for themselves and their families by migrating in search of economic opportunity, working long hours, and keeping their families and communities healthy, fed, and intact, they are routinely "othered" and excoriated in the press for trying to advance their lot in life by crossing the border. They are blamed for not having documentation, for not spending enough time at home raising their children because they are working long hours, for not paying taxes, and for their poverty wages. If undocumented migrants do seek government help, they can be defined as a "public charge," a designation that signals financial dependence on the state and that could prevent them from gaining authorization to stay in the United States. Being a public charge also has symbolic repercussions as it reinforces stereotypes of the lazy Mexican, who would rather take a siesta than work, or of Mexican migrants as "welfare magnets" having "anchor babies" so they can live off the generosity of the U.S. state.[56] The accusations against indigenous migrants point to their identities and cultures as the problem, as if earning poverty wages or preferring to work bent over is somehow a culturally or biologically defined attribute, rather than acknowledging that these factors are direct outcomes of their ineligibility for personhood in the United States.[57]

Despite their best attempts to keep their families stable, migrants are treated as illegal and worthless. They are punished by inhumane immigration policies that leave them to die in scorching deserts, to languish in U.S. detention centers, or, as in Perla's case, to suffer economic exploitation if they do make it to the United States. Instead of lauding their hard work, creativity, and resilience, their efforts at self-determination are instead framed as irresponsible and immoral, and they are regularly discriminated against and urged to return home. Paradoxically, however, for those that might find life in the United States too harsh and actually wish to return home, the costs and risks of going back have become prohibitive. The deadly U.S.-supported war on drugs, officially waged in Mexico between 2006–2018, which has killed at least 150,000 people to date, deterred many people from returning to Mexico.

State-sponsored violence and the rise of femicide in Oaxaca have forced people to rethink what going home would actually mean. Furthermore, people are reticent to leave given the escalating economic and physical costs associated with crossing the border back into the United States should they find conditions at home intolerable. Gaspar Rivera-Salgado sums up the dilemma: "The current enforcement policy is based on excluding them, through violence and jail at the border, and isolation and fear in their community. The idea is to make life so hard for them in the U.S. they'll have to leave. But where are they supposed to go?"[58] Increasingly strict border enforcement measures were more successful at keeping migrants in the United States than at keeping them out, leading to a situation of "forced permanence" for many.[59] Thus, while prevention through deterrence was meant to keep people out, it has actually had the opposite effect, leaving a "critical mass" of indigenous Oaxacans caught in limbo between two countries, subject to multiple forms of structural violence, and without rights or recognition.

Structural Determinants of Indigenous Health

The impacts that social, political, and economic inequities have on the body are often understood in terms of the social or structural determinants of health, or those environmental conditions that affect health, functioning, and quality-of-life outcomes and risks.[60] A quintessential indicator of social and economic vulnerability, health status often reflects inequitable living and working conditions.[61] As indigenous out-migration has increased, researchers have studied the social determinants of indigenous health in the United States. It is clear from this research that the embodied states of indigenous Mexicans are—given their extreme vulnerability as indigenous, migrant, poor, and often undocumented in the United States—overdetermined by the environments in which they live, work, and raise their families. In other words, their life outcomes are influenced by multiple forces, any one of which would be insufficient to account for their overall impact. The health of indigenous Oaxacans is a reflection of this convergence of forces.

Indigenous migrants are not without agency, yet in large part their health outcomes are both outside their personal control and beyond their biological or genetic makeup. They are the result of what medical anthropologists have called syndemic vulnerability.[62] Sarah Willen and her colleagues explain, "Syndemics emerge when two or more health conditions co-occur in environments of aggravated adversity and interact synergistically to yield worse health outcomes than each affliction would likely generate on its own."[63] Syndemic vulnerability occurs when these health conditions emerge and interact in populations experiencing significant adversity, thus creating a negative feedback loop between environmental factors, such as structural violence, and individual physical outcomes, such as illness, disease, and death. This dynamic can be described in the following way, "Beyond the notion of disease clustering in a location or population, and processes of biological synergism among co-dwelling pathogens, the term *syndemic* points to the determinant importance of *social conditions* in the health of individuals and populations."[64] For example, the rise of diabetes in Oaxaca's transnational population is the result of an emerging syndemic characterized by childhood undernutrition and infection, adult obesity and metabolic changes, and social conditions that have dismantled local food systems and propelled out-migration.[65]

Indigenous Oaxacans experience high levels of syndemic vulnerability. As described earlier, one of the strongest determinants of indigenous health is the racism they experience both in the United States and in Mexico.[66] Marginalized racial and ethnic groups in the United States confront greater health disparities than other groups. The hallmark text *Unequal Treatment: Confronting Racial and Ethnic Disparities in Healthcare*, produced by the Institute of Medicine in 2002, explains that "the majority of [health] studies . . . find that racial and ethnic disparities remain even after adjustment for socioeconomic differences and other healthcare access–related factors."[67] The study links health care disparities to historical patterns of legalized segregation and discrimination in the United States and argues that "much of American social and economic life remains ordered by race and ethnicity, with minorities disadvantaged relative to whites."[68] It also states that "minorities' experiences in the world outside of the healthcare practitioner's office are likely to affect their perceptions and responses in care settings."[69] These findings certainly hold true for indigenous Mexicans in California.

In his research with Triqui migrants in California and Washington State, physician-anthropologist Seth Holmes found that structural racism and anti-immigrant practices determine the poor working conditions, living conditions, and health of migrant workers.[70] Indigenous migrants are often called "Oaxaquito" or "Oaxaco" as a racial epithet.[71] So profound is this racism that one school district in Southern California prohibited the use of the terms "Oaxaquito" and "indito" in the school system.[72] Pervasive racism leads indigenous migrants to constantly be on their guard, as a Triqui interpreter explained, "Working in the field I saw a lot of discrimination. They call us Oaxaquita or Indios in the rows where I worked. I was always defending my people."[73]

Anti-indigenous sentiment not only results from the xenophobia of white Americans, however. It also comes from Mexican-origin mestizos. Interethnic tensions have been particularly palpable in Greenfield, California, where two anti-indigenous movements, Beautify Greenfield and Save Greenfield, were spearheaded by second- and third-generation children of Mexican migrants.[74] Arguing that "'invaders from the south' should be deported," members of Beautify Greenfield charged that "the new migrants ruined the town financially, 'destroyed' its school system, caused violent crimes and were part of gangs, which are pervasive in the Salinas Valley." In addition to blaming indigenous Oaxacans for the city's ills, they blamed Greenfield's Anglo police chief for favoritism and "extreme prejudice" against nonindigenous residents. The chief responded by saying that newly arriving immigrants have always been racialized and scapegoated by established communities in the United States: "During troubled economic times it's not unusual to blame the newcomers."[75] Against these charges of preferential treatment, he explained that indigenous Oaxacans are more often the victims than the perpetrators of crime in his city. Indeed, indigenous migrants frequently receive lower pay than their mestizo counterparts in the agricultural fields, and are often victims of robbery, especially just after payday.

Poverty is also a strong determinant of indigenous health, leading to the dismal living conditions they encounter as they move along the harvest seasons in both the United States and Mexico.[76] Journalist David Bacon has photographed many of the improvised arrangements indigenous Mexicans use for cheap or low-cost shelter.[77] In a series he did on Oaxacans living in Santa Rosa, California, he explains that "residents live in deprivation; they sleep on mattresses dragged into the bushes, cook on makeshift fireplaces in the reeds, and take shelter under tarps strung along trees.[78] There have also been reports of indigenous migrants sleeping in caves, makeshift plastic structures, and even holes underground.[79]

An example of dismal living conditions occurred in Malaga, a small community outside Fresno, California, where a group of over two hundred Mixtecs from the district of Juxtlahuaca were living in fifty-six trailers and cabins, surrounded by an oil dump, a scrap metal heap, a wrecking yard, a manure plant, and a propane business.[80] The trailer park had been designated decades earlier as a Superfund site, which meant that children living there played in soil contaminated with arsenic, mercury, lead, and an assortment of other chemicals.[81] This toxic environment led to a high rate of miscarriages and respiratory problems among the residents.[82] Scholars have pointed out that poverty goes hand in hand with such "environmental racism," a situation in which people of color live near or within environmentally hazardous or degraded environments.[83] Environmental racism is exacerbated by the abuses and discrimination of labor contractors and employers who take advantage of many workers' inability to speak fluent English or Spanish and subject them to exploitative and unhealthy conditions in the fields. More than once I heard from indigenous farmworkers that they were told by the *mayordomos* (managers) that the pesticides routinely sprayed on the fields where they were working were "medicine for the plants." There was never any mention that this "medicine" was toxic for humans nor that it contributed to miscarriages, breathing problems, and birth defects in farmworker children.[84]

Many of the health problems indigenous migrants face result from employment as farm laborers, as the following excerpt illustrates.[85]

Although many of the [agricultural] workers are young men who should be in the prime of health, many suffer from disorders associated with old age (e.g., hypertension, diabetes, obesity, high blood pressure, high cholesterol, and arthritis). In addition, more and more young families and single women with children are finding their way into the fields, compounding health care problems. Infectious diseases such as tuberculosis abound, and the incidence of depression, which manifests in myriad ways that are deleterious to health, increases the longer workers remain in the U.S.[86]

One study on indigenous farmworkers in Santa Barbara County found that headaches, sore muscles, and back problems were among the top symptoms reported by this group. The study documents that 38 percent of female respondents and 42 percent of males reported feeling ill after working in or near agricultural fields. Moreover, the study's authors note that health insurance access and utilization represent significant barriers to medical services for indigenous workers and their children.[87] Medical anthropologist Bonnie Bade expands this perspective by explaining, "Among the barriers to adequate health care for Mixtec families in California are transportation problems, profound language differences, aid qualifications requirements, illiteracy, lack of documentation of legal residency, differing cultural and medical concepts held by practitioners and patients, extensive filling out of forms, and inappropriate scheduling demands."[88]

In an unpublished study on the health conditions of Mexican indigenous farmworkers, Bade found that almost half of those surveyed had dental problems, about 10 percent had respiratory problems, 44 percent suffered back pain, almost one-fifth had stomach pain, 30 percent suffered eye problems, and 20 percent had experienced an occupation-related injury. In addition, respondents reported other conditions, such as hepatitis (16 percent), skin conditions and allergies (16 percent), diabetes (10 percent), tuberculosis (6 percent), and anemia (6 percent). Survey respondents worked only sporadically, and their working conditions included exposure to harsh environmental conditions and pesticides.[89] All of this leads to high levels of stress and anxiety, which have been linked to alcohol abuse, domestic violence, and depression.[90] Indeed, every one of the community health workers interviewed for this book cited depression as the primary health issue affecting indigenous migrants.

Unfortunately, migrants face multiple barriers—including language, transportation, documentation, and the ability to take time off work without being fired—that prevent them from accessing the services that could help alleviate these troubles. Added to this is the fact that there are few if any mental health services available in farmworker communities, nor are there many programs that deal with domestic violence prevention. This means, as more than one health promoter explained to me, that when men feel depressed they take it out on their wives, who, for fear of interacting with the police or being kicked out by their husbands, *se aguantan* (they put up with it).

The structural violence that indigenous Mexicans face affects their ability to afford necessities such as food. In a study conducted in the San Joaquin Valley of California, Katherine Moos found that among her Mixtec focus group participants, 93 percent (25 of 27) had experienced food insecurity in 2007, and 89 percent (24 of 27) reported that "sometimes we don't have enough to eat."[91] Indigenous migrants work in the breadbasket of the world, bringing healthy fruits and vegetables to our tables so that we might flourish, yet they and their children suffer.[92] Such a paradox signals a dynamic in which multiple generations of indigenous Mexicans trade their long-term health for economic and biological survival. Given this, it is no wonder that Seth Holmes argues that structural violence is so harmful to the body that in the end it has the same injurious effects as a stabbing or shooting.[93]

Migrant Resistance: A Binational Effort

In the face of these pathologies of power, indigenous migrants have adopted diverse methods for contesting their social and physical suffering.[94] Migration has offered an immediate solution to violence in their communities of origin, while cross-border activism has represented a more sustained and important counterforce to the violence and discrimination they experience. As Gaspar Rivera-Salgado argues, "Indigenous migrants, far from becoming passive victims of the discriminatory and exploitative conditions they face on both sides of the Mexico–US border, have responded in a highly creative way, building cross-border political organizations that make collective action possible in both their communities of origin and those established along their migratory circuit."[95]

Rivera-Salgado's sentiments have been echoed by Odilia Romero, a trilingual Zapotec woman, interpreter, and binational activist living in Los Angeles, who insists that indigenous Mexicans are not poor, helpless, or needy, but strong, organized, powerful, and creative. As she explained during a speech she gave at Cornell University, and cited at the outset of this chapter, "Indigenous people are thinkers, we're intellectuals, and we participate in decisions that affect our lives. We aren't just here to pick your strawberries."[96] Indeed, first-generation indigenous activists have engaged in community organizing, held public protests, dialogued directly with high-level politicians (including Mexican presidents), made public statements, offered counternarratives to anti-immigrant discourses, and taught indigenous migrants their rights—all while proposing and affirming a unified indigenous identity.[97] Second-generation indigenous youth are continuing this tradition by building youth leadership, teaching indigenous languages and traditions, and organizing for social change and social justice.[98] Female indigenous farmworkers also organize for health, leadership, and female empowerment, speaking out against the injustices they have faced.[99]

All of these positive strategies focus on obtaining political rights and cultural recognition. Silvia Jacquelina Ramírez Romero, who has written a book about the history of indigenous Mexican activism, explains, "Their identity as indigenous not only translates into specific strategies but also into a permanent orientation toward the re-creation of their culture thereby giving life and meaning to their actions."[100] Affirmative cultural practices complement civic engagement and are an integral part of indigenous resistance in the United States. Indigenous Mexican migrant activists recuperated indigenous languages, customs, and dress. They also teach indigenous dances and indigenous recipes. Both affirming and re-creating indigenous cultural identity in the face of economic, political, and social forces that degrade the health and well-being of indigenous migrants has been a core project of indigenous migrant activism. La Agencia was an outgrowth of this activism.

La Agencia emerged from the struggles of several different organizations fighting against the discrimination, marginalization, and violence facing indigenous groups in the Mixtec, Zapotec, and Triqui regions of Oaxaca, Mexico, beginning in the 1970s.[101] As Oaxaca experienced increasing out-migration of indigenous people, especially Mixtecs, to other Mexican states, such as Sinaloa, Sonora, and Baja California, and eventually across the border to California, the indigenous movement followed.[102] In these states, migrant workers fought for labor rights and continued their struggle against the exploitation of indigenous Oaxacans. A binational indigenous social movement was born on October 5, 1991, in Los Angeles, California, in the context of mobilization efforts across the hemisphere to signal 500 years of resistance by indigenous people, whose genocide and ethnocide were being erased in the 1992 celebrations glorifying the "discovery" of America by Christopher Columbus.[103]

The creation of this binational organization brought several Mixtec and Zapotec organizations under one umbrella to address problems confronting indigenous Mexicans as both workers and migrants. The problems they identified reflect those outlined earlier in the chapter, including the violation of human rights, violence, discrimination, racial offenses, social marginalization, extortion by the police, and labor abuses. The goal of this organization was to defend the human rights and labor rights of indigenous migrants in California, as well as to establish a permanent communication network among the different organizations in order to support projects in their communities of origin.

Over time, the organization changed as some participants dropped out and others joined. It eventually solidified into the Binational Indigenous Resistance Movement (BIRM) and continued to focus on defending the rights of indigenous workers, supporting communities of origin, and confronting problems having to do with migration. Central to their struggles for human rights has been the use of indigenous culture as the basis for leadership and as an expression of indigenous people's dignity. Events such as an annual basketball tournament and the campaign against 500 years of colonization inform the organization's political and economic goals of autonomy and self-determination.

Structural Violence and the Birth of La Agencia

Shortly after consolidating their organization, the governing body of BIRM realized that they also needed a way to address the ongoing, everyday problems faced by indigenous migrants. This led to the birth of La Agencia in 1993. La Agencia was created in response to the profound structural violence that indigenous Mexicans have suffered but also in recognition of the fact that they were not helpless in the face of this suffering. They could act to help their people and to affirm their dignity and rights in both the United States and Mexico. La Agencia was developed as a conduit for direct services and civic education for indigenous Mexicans and as a fiscal sponsor for BIRM.

The relationship that developed between BIRM and La Agencia has been mutually beneficial and complementary. La Agencia serves as a fiscal agent through which funding for BIRM's activities in Mexico and California is funneled. In turn, La Agencia serves BIRM's membership base in California by providing interpretation services and educational workshops on health, leadership, and civic participation. BIRM focuses primarily on political organizing and rights education, whereas La Agencia concentrates on providing indigenous migrants throughout California with access to social services and information. Although linked ideologically and in constant communication, the two organizations are autonomous and have their own governing bodies, though there is some overlap in their leadership and membership. In the last few years, both organizations have engaged in a "self-reflection" process and realized that leadership development, gender equity, and, most recently, the incorporation of youth need to be central components in their strategies. They are also both committed to activities that maintain indigenous Oaxacan culture, and they work together on events such as an annual Guelaguetza celebration, which is centered on indigenous dances and food.

Building on this strong foundation, La Agencia has grown over the years and currently has programs in several regions throughout California, including the San Joaquin Valley, the Salinas Valley, Santa Barbara County, and Los Angeles. Their main office is located in the Central Valley. In addition, they are affiliated with offices in Oaxaca and Baja California, Mexico, through their relationship with BIRM. La Agencia's mission is to implement programs that stimulate civic participation and the economic, social, and cultural development of indigenous communities. Their vision is to achieve the well-being, equity, and self-determination of indigenous communities. The IHP is one of the core programs for implementing this mission and achieving this vision.

El Proyecto de Salud Indígena: A Bidirectional Strategy

La Agencia's health promotion work began in 1997 as a collaborative effort with a farmworker women's organization. The original project, Farmworker Women United (Trabajadoras Agrícolas Unidas), provided indigenous migrant women with health information about breast cancer, diabetes, pesticides in the fields, and domestic violence, among other themes. It also developed female leadership so indigenous women could play a meaningful role in the democratic decision-making processes of the organization. In 1998, La Agencia took over full control of the project; it continued to foster leadership for women and to hold educational health workshops and events on women's health in Fresno, Kern, Madera, and Merced Counties, as well as in Los Angeles, Santa Barbara, and Santa Cruz.

In 2001, La Agencia reduced the geographic area in which they provided services but expanded their target audience to include the whole family and not just indigenous women. They also expanded to work with Zapotecs living in Los Angeles. By this time, many more women had become involved in La Agencia's services and activities. This new iteration of the program had several goals, including identifying indigenous communities and their needs, providing disease-prevention workshops, conducting basic health exams, and organizing health fairs. At the same time, they provided cultural sensitivity workshops to social service providers. As part of the cultural sensitivity trainings, the organization developed a guidebook on Oaxacan culture and organized conferences about the use of indigenous, or "traditional," medicine.

The "Oaxacan Culture: Cultural Competence Guidebook" an unpublished resource guide authored by La Agencia staff and a number of their academic allies, details many aspects of indigenous lifestyle, including healing practices. It explains that indigenous health beliefs and practices, commonly known as traditional or indigenous medicine, are thousands of years old. Indigenous approaches to health reflect strong ties to Mother Earth and differ significantly from allopathic or Western medicine insofar as indigenous perceptions of illness and health are closely interwoven with religion and social relations. The guidebook tells its readers that indigenous Oaxacans practice traditional medicine wherever they migrate within and outside of Mexico, often supplementing it with clinical care. Yet, because of their use of traditional medicine they have faced discrimination from mestizos, who call them witches, sorcerers or *brujos*, a term that belittles the importance and efficacy of the medicine they practice. Despite this discrimination, indigenous communities are very proud to have an in-depth knowledge of herbs and the gifts nature provides. This pride was expressed by an indigenous healer:

> We continue and will continue to use traditional medicine wherever we live because it has always cured us. Often the medicines that are available in the pharmacy are made of the same ingredients that we use to cure ourselves. We will also continue to use our medicine because many indigenous migrants don't have health insurance such as Medi-Cal and clinical visits in the United States are too expensive for us. What is good about traditional medicine is that we do not need an appointment. Any day or hour we can go get healed or even heal ourselves in our own homes. We can prepare our own remedies. When we go to be healed by a traditional medicine doctor, he/she cures more than the illnesses that are affecting us in the moment. Another benefit is that our families can be present during the healing. At the end of the healing we feel good, rested in our bodies and our spirits because we have reencountered ourselves and we know the cause of our illness.

The millennia-old traditions of indigenous healing are one of the ways that indigenous peoples combat the pathologies of power they have experienced. Indigenous medicine thus functions as a collective response to assaults on indigenous identity, society, and culture. This does not mean, however, that indigenous Oaxacans are not open to Western medicine or to clinical care. It simply means that they have a more copious healing repertoire than those who subscribe exclusively to allopathic medicine and that they look for cures to what ails them in places beyond the health care market.

Train-the-Trainer

From 2004 to 2007, the IHP was again funded to conduct work in Fresno, Kern, Merced, Monterey, and Tulare. This iteration of the program continued to provide all of the services it had been offering, including one-on-one help to indigenous migrants in navigating the social service, education, and health systems. Several components changed, however. The program launched a community health worker, or promotora, model, which operates from a "train-the-trainer" approach so that, as I was told by an employee of La Agencia, "the health workers themselves take responsibility for helping their communities regarding questions of health and social services." The train-the-trainer model is based on adult learning theory, which states that people who train others remember 90 percent of what they teach, and on the diffusion of innovation theory, which states that people adopt new information through trusted social networks.[104]

Training the trainers (who will, in turn, train more trainers) is promoted as a cost-effective and culturally competent model for involving people in the social and political issues that affect their lives. It operates from an assets-based approach that recognizes the knowledge and experience of the participants and builds on these strengths to foster leadership. La Agencia's goal was to expose as many indigenous community members as possible to leadership training so that the audience for the lessons it provided on health issues could grow exponentially. The model was highly successful because it drew from the social capital of La Agencia's staff and built on the strong social networks that exist within the indigenous migrant communities throughout California. It was also successful because it used the cultural capital of the indigenous women who worked as promotoras to convey the information to program participants in culturally and linguistically relevant ways.

The other change that occurred during this period was the explicit inclusion of interpretation services. Contrary to what many people think, there is no language called "Oaxacan," and each indigenous group from Oaxaca has its own language with distinct dialects. Indigenous migrants need help accessing health and other social services in their own language because they are fearful of being misunderstood and of being discriminated against for not speaking English or Spanish. As one of the health workers for the IHP explained, "When you don't speak the language that is being spoken around you, simple things are difficult to accomplish. Even calling the doctor is scary." Figuring out which language and dialect is being spoken by a patient can be tricky, but the stakes are high: indigenous migrants have faced countless barriers navigating U.S. society because of the language differences, which create difficulty communicating with landlords and employers or make it impossible to speak with doctors, nurses, teachers, or other professionals with whom they need to interact on a regular basis.[105] Further, few indigenous migrants know that they have the right to access services from government-funded programs in their language, which means they fail to demand the interpretation services they should be receiving by law.

The lack of language accessibility has caused misunderstandings with serious consequences. Several of the examples I learned of while conducting research for this book included a Triqui man who was institutionalized for years in Oregon for not speaking or understanding Spanish. He was eventually released, but only after the mental health professionals learned that the language he spoke was a recognized indigenous language and not gibberish. In another example, Mixtec parents were blamed for "trying to kill their child" and were incarcerated in Fresno, California. It turned out that they, like many indigenous language speakers, acted like they understood what was being told to them in Spanish by answering "Sí" to all of the doctor's questions, but in actuality they did not fully understand the doctor's instructions and did the opposite of what was asked of them. To avoid these misunderstandings La Agencia staff teaches indigenous language speakers that they have the right to interpretation. The staff also provide interpretation services themselves and train others to be interpreters.

To summarize, the main objectives of the IHP during this period were to (1) provide health information to the indigenous community through workshops and health fairs; (2) help indigenous migrants navigate the social service system by filling out documents and providing interpretation services; (3) employ the promotora model to train indigenous promotoras; and (4) use workshops, presentations, and a cultural guidebook to educate service providers about the presence and culture of indigenous Mexicans in California and their use of indigenous medicine.

Through this path-breaking work La Agencia made every effort to help indigenous migrants access much-needed health services while at the same time working with providers to make those services more accessible. In doing this, they set an example for other indigenous migrant organizations in the United States to follow, partnered with migrant-supporting organizations in California and across the country, and became a beacon of hope for newly arriving migrant families. Most importantly, the staff of the IHP continued a long tradition of indigenous activism by actively working to reshape the violent social and political structures informing indigenous lives in the United States and Mexico.

Conclusion

As this chapter has shown, indigenous Mexicans face significant barriers to their health and well-being, both in Mexico and in the United States. In response to these barriers, they have exhibited creative and pragmatic solutions for changing violent structures and helping those affected by them. They have done this by building pan-ethnic indigenous social movements that promote grassroots activism, through political lobbying in both the United States and Mexico, and, as Perla's presentation exemplifies, by telling the public about their lives using the Latin American tradition of *testimonio* and, most significantly, by demanding their rights. These forms of indigenous migrant activism are rooted in a long history of indigenous resistance to oppression and discrimination, and they build on indigenous values of collective self-determination, autonomy, mutual aid, and indigenous sovereignty.

Indigenous migrants have also tried to counter structural violence by building institutions of their own. La Agencia is an example of this. Recognizing that political change is slow and that people's everyday needs had to be met in the meantime, they developed a nonprofit agency to address those immediate needs and to serve as a fiscal sponsor for their political activism. Because La Agencia's leadership is made up of indigenous Mexican migrants who understood and had themselves experienced the unhealthy effects of structural violence, one of the programs they developed was the IHP. The IHP went through several iterations in accordance with the needs of the community, the available funding, and the objectives of the staff and its board of directors. Nevertheless, a core focus was always the dual emphasis on indigenous health and indigenous culture.

Taken together, La Agencia's efforts can be understood as an exercise in "structural competency." Defined as "medicine for the inequalities that make us sick," structural competency is "the trained ability to discern how a host of issues defined clinically as symptoms, attitudes or diseases (e.g., depression, hypertension, obesity smoking, medication 'non-compliance,' trauma, psychosis) also represent the downstream implications of a number of upstream decisions about such matters as health care and food delivery systems, zoning laws, urban and rural infrastructures, medicalization, or even about the very definitions of illness and health." As health researchers have begun to argue, upstream factors play a much greater role than genetics, access to health care, or individual decisions in shaping individual and population health outcomes.[106] This means that changing those things that occur "upstream" will go much farther in improving health outcomes than genetic technologies, a health care system overhaul, or individual behavioral changes ever would. La Agencia's staff recognized this when they wrote the "Oaxacan Culture: Cultural Competence Guidebook":

> Given the complexity of the challenges this group faces, advocacy efforts for indigenous health need to address both the conditions and the policies which negatively impact their ability to care for themselves and their

families. Two areas in particular where policy reform could bring positive changes in the health status of indigenous Mexicans in the U.S. are immigration and health care. Current laws which restrict access to health coverage based on citizenship status contribute to health disparities and infringe upon the human right to health care that all people regardless of documentation are entitled to.[107]

This focus on policy change to mitigate health inequities and ensure human rights resonates with an understanding of health as social justice. Indeed, this understanding always informed La Agencia's program development, including the IHP. What its architects did not account for, however, was the ways that the health work they were doing was informed by and, in many ways promoting, the neoliberal ideologies and policies that they were resisting. As chapter 3 shows, although the La Agencia staff understood their health programming to be operating in the service of a social justice and human rights agenda, and against structural violence, the programming may at the same time have been working at cross-purposes with those very same objectives. Indeed, just as indigenous political repertoires, healing practices, and cultural norms have shifted over time and across space as Oaxacans increasingly migrate to the United States, so too have the meanings and purposes of health promotion.

Chapter 3

The "Mexican Model" of Health

Examining the Travels and Translations of Health Promotion

**Health promotion is not apolitical, rather it is
an explicitly, politically orientated activity.**

"Ni Tengo Carro"

I walked into the large, first-floor conference room of a historical building in the downtown of a large, Central Valley city. Eight Mixtec women were seated in a row behind a long table listening attentively to a presentation on child car seat safety. Since I had arrived a bit late and there were no more seats at the table, I pulled up a chair just behind them. A female employee from the county health department was describing proper installation procedures and the California laws that apply to child car seat use. As she manipulated the buckles and belts on the child seat, explaining in Spanish the use of each, none of the eight women moved or spoke. At the end of her demonstration, the presenter inquired as to whether any of the women had any questions. Everyone remained silent. Seeing that there were no comments from the group, the Mixtec *promotora* (community health worker) who had arranged the presentation stood up and thanked her while the health department representative began to collect her materials. At that moment of transition, one of the eight women turned to her neighbor shaking her head and, in a voice just above a whisper, said, "ni tengo carro" (I don't even have a car).

I begin with this story because it was the first of many health education workshops I was to attend during my field research. I recount it here because it is emblematic of the kinds of disconnects that I witnessed repeatedly as health workers sought to give advice to indigenous migrants on a variety of health and lifestyle issues. As this example shows, the barriers to accessing health information for indigenous Mexican migrants extend beyond the cultural and linguistic challenges experienced by indigenous program participants. That is, it is not just because many indigenous migrants do not speak fluent Spanish or because they have unique health beliefs or cultural practices that they have difficulty making use of the health information and services provided to them. Rather, it is because that information and those services often do not account for their social position and economic status, as demonstrated by the woman who has no need for a car seat given that she has neither a car nor a driver's license because of her undocumented status.[1]

These kinds of mismatches, in which a particular kind of informed, middle-class health consumer is both assumed and proposed as the ideal also extend into the clinic, contributing to the marginalization and embodied vulnerability of indigenous migrants. For example, one of La Agencia's Mixtec promotoras explained to me that when she took her son, who was wheezing a lot, to the clinic, he was diagnosed with asthma. She was instructed to go buy some medicine to help him with his breathing. When she got to the pharmacy she gave the cashier her son's name and they charged her for his medicine. When she opened the bag at home she found that instead of the bottle of liquid medicine she expected to find there was an oval-shaped plastic apparatus (a diffuser that helps the child inhale the medicine), a red plastic container with a hole down the middle (the inhaler), and a metal cartridge (the asthma medicine). She had no idea what any of them were for nor how they went together. In her case, like the car seat situation, there was a mismatch between the idealized health consumer, whose health care decisions and purchases are assumed to be informed and deliberate, and the actual health consumer, whose practices and understandings are often influenced by a variety of factors, understandings, and sources of information.

This mismatch between the ideal and the real health care recipient is consequential. As Bonnie Bade has pointed out in her research with Mixtecs in California, the assumption of a universal health subject is not only false, it is alienating. "Expensive biomedical treatments, lack of health insurance, language barriers, transportation problems, and cultural differences concerning illness causation and treatment combine to marginalize Mixtec families from the mainstream biomedical health care culture."[2] At stake in this disjuncture for many migrant families are both prolonged illnesses and expensive hospitalizations for conditions that could have been prevented. Families may be left with devastating medical debt, a reduced ability to work, and, in extreme cases, death. Thus "access" and "utilization" of health care information, services, and products are not just about availability, they are also about a biomedical health care culture that, despite its professed concern for cultural competence, fails to fully understand the complex structural differences that actually make the difference when it comes to health care use. By focusing almost exclusively on patient culture, and by failing to acknowledge that health care systems have their own cultures replete with values, languages, dialects, customs, clothing, and traditions that interact with patients' cultures, health workers rarely recognize the ways that the culture of health is itself exacerbating health care problems and inaccessibility for many. Indeed, one of the problematic assumptions prevalent in U.S. health care systems is the idea that patients are the only ones whose culture counts.

Health workers also often fail to see how their best attempts at being culturally competent reinforce harmful and simplistic stereotypes about patients. For example, "Mexican culture" is often cited as the source of health promotion programs developed for Mexican migrants in California despite the fact that this "culture" is made up of many cultures. There are over sixty-two distinct indigenous groups in Mexico, each with its own language, dialect, traditions, and customs. Further, there have been multiple generations of indigenous Mexicans who have migrated to or been born in the United States. This means that indigenous families are often trilingual (indigenous language, Spanish, and English), and they embrace a variety of customs and norms, some from the United States, some from their communities of origin, and some from other places or people they have encountered from different backgrounds or nations. For example, I regularly saw Oaxacan farmworkers eating at the Chinese buffet and indigenous children playing Super Mario in English on their Nintendo DS. The idea of a "Mexican culture" therefore creates more confusion than it resolves.

Nevertheless, the idea of Mexican culture pervaded the health programs and policies I studied. When I asked why health promotion had become such an important focus of social service programs for Mexican migrants, the response I most often received was about cultural tradition. "It's what they do in Mexico" I was told by Joaquin Santamaria, the architect of a $25 million agricultural worker's health initiative in California. Joaquin's sentiments were echoed in my first meeting with the former executive director of La Agencia, Ramon Garcia, a Mixtec man from the Oaxacan town of San Miguel Cuevas. Ramon explained that the Indigenous Health Project was modeled on the "Mexican model" of health promotion, which he was familiar with in his home state of Oaxaca. "It's what they know in the villages back home, so we decided to do it here, too."

Because health promotion was seen to be rooted in Mexican cultural tradition, it was also assumed to be culturally competent. For example, as we sat in his high-rise office in the same downtown where the car seat workshop was held, Ramon explained that La Agencia's health workshops were culturally competent both because they mirrored the kinds of programs that he and others had experienced back home in Mexico and because they were delivered by indigenous migrants who spoke the indigenous languages of the program participants (mostly Mixtec and Triqui), who often had migrated from the same Oaxacan villages as those they were speaking to.

The programs that I observed were in fact delivered in relevant languages by people with familiar faces wearing traditional clothing, but the content of those programs did not always reflect the values, practices, and experiences of the indigenous program participants or even the experiences of the promotoras themselves. The car seat example described earlier highlights this mismatch. In other words, the culture of health within the Indigenous Health Project did not always mirror the cultural values and practices of indigenous Mexican migrants as they expressed these values and practices to me and to the broader public (as discussed in chapter 5). To the extent the program participants were from diverse ethnic and linguistic backgrounds, geographic communities, and generations, their beliefs and understandings did not reflect one homogeneous "Mexican" or "indigenous" culture. Because of this diversity, there was often a mismatch between the assumed and the actual indigenous health subject being targeted by La Agencia's health programming. This observed disjuncture led me to ask why La Agencia was supporting and promoting versions of health that their program participants often did not understand or need, as in the car seat example. In order to make sense of this mismatch, this chapter illuminates what other cultures are at work in the Indigenous Health Project.

The Flavor of the Month

As discussed in chapter 2, recognition of the embodied effects of structural violence in indigenous migrant communities goes some way toward explaining why health promotion is deemed so important. La Agencia creatively uses health promotion as a way to mitigate the effects of inequitable social and political arrangements and to advocate for the cultural and biological survival of indigenous peoples. In this way, health promotion facilitates a social justice agenda that addresses the very real and pressing needs of La Agencia's program participants. From this perspective, health is used to empower indigenous Mexican communities not only to survive but to thrive in a context of great uncertainty and precarity.

The idea that health promotion is a "Mexican" cultural tradition also adds some explanatory value. It is true that Mexico has had several iterations of health promotion programs, discussed later in the chapter, that have utilized promotoras to deliver health information and services to poor, rural communities. These programs have been critiqued, however, for promoting market citizenship under the guise of empowerment.[3] This critique of the neoliberal underpinnings of health promotion gets us a little closer to another of the explanations for why health was chosen as the focus of so many social service programs for migrants, including La Agencia's.

When I asked an experienced community organizer employed by the multimillion-dollar agricultural initiative why health promotion, rather than another form of political work such as grassroots organizing or political lobbying, had become the mechanism for empowering farmworker communities to confront structural violence he replied, "because health is the flavor of the month." When asked to elaborate, he explained that there was significant funding for health at a time when barriers to health care access were growing in the United States and health care services were increasingly managed in and through the market. Nonprofits that were in the business of providing social support and services were rapidly retooling so they could access that funding. Because social service workers and the organizations they work for relied on grant funding, the health programs they developed did not challenge the mandates of their economic benefactors, but rather sought to creatively implement them. Nonprofits need grant money to survive and because there were a lot of grants for health at a time when health care in the United States was shifting to managed care, health promotion became "the flavor of the month." Given this, a direct feedback loop was established between the economic survival of nonprofits and the biological survival of those they served. The more health they promoted, the more they could bring in institution-sustaining funding, and the more health they could promote. This feedback loop was sustained by a broader dynamic in which health philanthropists supported "self-help poverty action," rather than radical structural change, in order to maintain the status quo. Not only did this protect the economic and political interests of philanthropic organizations while boosting their moral capital, it also served to obscure the harmful relationship between agricultural modes of production and the moral, behavioral and now entrepreneurial responsibilities of impoverished farmworkers.[4]

Taken together, the structural vulnerability of indigenous Mexicans, the cultural relevance of the "Mexican model," and the comment about flavor of the

month explain why the health focus was adopted as an activist strategy for helping indigenous migrants in California. This comprehensive explanation does
not, however, account for why individual behavioral change based on a combination of biomedical and public health science became the basis for the Indigenous Health Project. As described in chapter 2, indigenous peoples have
millennial traditions they have drawn on to promote and protect their health
so why not promote those? In order to understand why this particular version
of health became the focus of La Agencia's efforts, it is necessary to take a closer
look at the history of the Mexican model of health promotion and the kinds of
political economic forces that have influenced its travels and translations across
time and place. A close examination reveals that the Mexican model itself has
political and economic origins that start well before this model arrived in Mexico
and that, while these origins were at the beginning aligned with the kinds of
politics focused on social justice and equity that La Agencia is invested in, the
model changed over time and came to stand for something quite different from
its original intent. Namely, it started out as an endeavor to foster social justice
and empower poor communities across the globe by advocating government
programs that support "health for all." It ended up as an activity that encourages "all for health" by pushing the poor to take added responsibility for their
health and their well-being in and through the market.

Indeed, as one community health worker optimistically explained to me
when I asked him what his goals were for the health workshops he delivered,
"The point is to empower communities, to make them feel that they own the
problem." Within community health circles, this idea of "ownership" is meant
to reflect agency and empowerment in health programs. Yet such ownership too
often involves holding vulnerable populations responsible for changing the
structural circumstances that are making them vulnerable while also making
them accountable to the philanthropists who support them. This feeling of moral
responsibility for community health reflected the dynamic at work in the
multimillion-dollar agricultural health worker program that was being implemented throughout California during my period of fieldwork. Community leadership groups made up of farmworkers were created throughout the state for
the purposes of confronting powerful agricultural growers. Unsurprisingly, the
community leaders felt compelled to implement their mandates because they
had been funded to do so even as they were terrified by what this would mean
in the long term for their jobs. These vulnerable farmworkers not only had to
take ownership for improving the health of their communities within this initiative, they were also responsible for making the nonprofits they worked with

and the funders who supported them feel and look good while not offending the billion-dollar agricultural industry they worked in.

Drawing from the material conditions that permit the travels and translations of health promotion, including conferences, charters, documents, human bodies, scientific expertise, public and private programs, and the like, this chapter shows that, contrary to the idea of a culturally relevant and stable Mexican model, the technical and material methods of health promotion carry along with them changing ethical and political orientations to the body and health. These orientations have, over time, come to reflect neoliberal ideas about how subjects should be governed, and should govern themselves, in and through health norms and practices. It is the promotion of these embodied norms and practices that inform the Indigenous Health Project in California.

A Brief History of Health Promotion

The first global conference on health promotion was held in Ottawa, Canada, in 1986, during which thirty-nine countries came together to discuss the growing need for primary health care. Organized "as a response to growing expectations for a new public health movement around the world," the Ottawa conference proposed health promotion as the answer to global health issues.[5] This gathering resulted in the "Ottawa Charter," which has been characterized as the "Bible" of health promotion because it represented "the ultimate ideal and vision of how the goal of health should be obtained through actions at various levels: global, national, community and individual."[6]

The "Ottawa Charter" defines health promotion as "the process of enabling people to increase control over, and to improve their health." Accordingly, it states the following: "To reach a state of complete, physical, mental, and social well-being, an individual or group must be able to identify and realize aspirations, to satisfy needs, and to change or cope with the environment. . . . People cannot achieve their fullest health potential unless they are able to take control of those things which determine their health. This must apply equally to men and women."[7] Unlike more targeted approaches, the Charter takes a broad definition of health and "following in the footsteps of the best traditions of public health and social medicine and making full use of the research on the impact of social factors on health, it links the production of health explicitly to 'prerequisites for health' such as peace, income, housing and—most important—defines health promotion as a process of empowerment and capacity building."[8]

As the Charter states, health promotion was conceptualized as a strategy for ensuring "Health for All by the Year 2000." This proposition built on the progress made through the Declaration on Primary Health Care developed at the International Conference on Primary Health Care held in Alma Ata, Kazakhstan, USSR, in 1978; the World Health Organization's Targets for All document; and the debate at the World Health Assembly on intersectoral action for health.[9] Of these documents, the Declaration of Alma Ata was perhaps the most significant precursor to the Ottawa Charter outlining a global health agenda based on primary health care services.

The goal of health for all as established in the Declaration on Primary Health Care, was that "a main social target of all governments, international organizations and the whole world community in the coming decades should be the attainment by all peoples of the world by the year 2000 of a level of health that will permit them to lead a socially and economically productive life."[10] Some of the goals set were that at least 5 percent of gross national product should be spent on health; at least 90 percent of children should have a weight for their age that corresponds to the reference values; safe water should be available in the home or within a fifteen-minute walking distance, and adequate sanitary facilities should be available in the home or immediate vicinity; people should have access to trained personnel for attending pregnancy or childbirth; and child care should be available for up to one year of age.[11]

The Declaration on Primary Health Care was based on a joint publication by UNICEF and the World Health Organization (WHO) in 1975 entitled *Alternative Approaches to Meeting Basic Health Needs in Developing Countries*. According to Marcos Cueto, that jointly authored report underlined the shortcomings of traditional vertical programs concentrating on specific diseases and criticized the assumption that the expansion of "Western" medical systems would meet the needs of the common people in "developing" countries.[12] It also examined successful approaches to primary health care in Bangladesh, China, Cuba, India, Niger, Nigeria, Tanzania, Venezuela, and Yugoslavia in order to identify the key factors in their success. As stated in the Declaration of Alma Ata, primary health care is "essential health care . . . made universally accessible to individuals and families in the community through their full participation and at a cost the community and country can afford. . . . . It forms an integral part of the country's health system, of which it is the central function and main focus, and of the overall social and economic development of the community."[13] With the adoption of primary health care at Alma Ata, the global discussion shifted from how to provide cost-effective primary *medical* care to a focus on primary health care, which entailed engaging people in their own health through the prevention of illness and disease rather than waiting for them to show up already sick at the hospital or doctor's office. Primary health care is not the equivalent of primary medical care; its scope is much broader and its orientation is different insofar as it moves away from having medical authorities and hospitals as the first line of intervention once illness strikes and toward engaging all community members in preventing illness from occurring. As Kaprio explains, "The co-operation of social workers, teachers, local industrial leaders, trade union groups, transport authorities, and of course the local political authorities—that is, all who can influence people's health at a local level—is a crucial requirement for primary health care. Finally and most important are the people themselves as individuals, families and groups of interested people. These may include groups concerned with the environment, road safety, accident prevention or the problems of alcohol and drug abuse, consumer associations, such as those for diabetics or the parents of mentally retarded children."[14] He explains that this list is not comprehensive but should serve as an example of how complex a community's network of primary health care activities can be. Given this, the global goal of health for all as conceptualized within the primary health care framework simultaneously implies "all for health."

The Declaration, like the Charter that followed eight years later, linked global peace to global health, while urging governments, WHO, UNICEF, other international organizations, multilateral and bilateral agencies, nongovernmental organizations, funding agencies, all health workers, and the whole world community to support national and international commitments to primary health care, and to channel increased technical and financial support to it, especially in developing countries. This founding document based its definition of health on that used by WHO since the 1940s, defining it broadly as a state of complete physical, mental, and social well-being and not merely the absence of illness or infirmity. It also defined health as a fundamental human right, the attainment of which "is a most important world-wide social goal whose realization requires the action of many other social and economic sectors in addition to the health sector."[15]

Asserting that inequality in health status between people in developed and developing countries is politically, socially, and economically unacceptable and is therefore of common concern to all countries, the Declaration claims that the promotion and protection of the health of the people is essential to sustained economic and social development and contributes to a better quality of life and to world peace. The Declaration posits the attainment of health through primary health care as a right of the people whose duty it is to participate individually and collectively in the planning and implementation of health care. It also claims that it is the responsibility of governments to provide adequate health and social measures and to do so in conjunction with other pertinent sectors while also requiring and promoting maximum community and individual self-reliance and participation in the planning, organization, operation, and control of primary health care.

Through this document, the global imperative to health was also linked to the global imperative to development and modernization for it was understood that an unhealthy population was not a productive one and that modernization would continue to elude those countries that were wanting or needing to be "developed," but whose population was not in top form. Insofar as global differences in wealth among "developed" and "developing" countries caused political and military conflicts, the imperative to health as an economic development strategy was also conceptualized as a political panacea, hence its connection within the Declaration and subsequent charters, such as that adopted in 1986 at Ottawa and most recently in 2005 at the 6th Global Conference on Health Promotion in Bangkok, Thailand, to peace, human security, and global governance.[16]

The Declaration of Alma Ata was followed six years later by the publication of a report written in 1974 by Marc Lalonde, then minister of health for Canada. This document entitled "A New Perspective on the Health of Canadians: A Working Document," was also instrumental in shaping the agenda of the Ottawa Charter. At the core of Lalonde's report was the argument that individuals were hurting themselves and the economic strength of the Canadian nation through their behaviors. The behaviors in question had to do with what Lalonde called "counter-forces that constitute the dark side of economic progress."[17] These included, "environmental pollution, city living, habits of indolence, the abuse of alcohol, tobacco and drugs, and eating patterns which put the pleasing of the senses above the needs of the human body."[18] He argued that based on a study of the causes of early mortality and hospital morbidity (i.e., those cases in which someone was treated in the hospital), Canadians between the ages of one and seventy were dying mainly from vehicle accidents, heart disease, other accidents, respiratory diseases and lung cancer, and suicide. These were the same factors that caused the highest number of hospitalizations in 1970, the year for which the data were collected. Based on these findings, he concluded that self-imposed risk and environmental factors were at fault and that the organized health care system would do little more than serve as a catchment net for the victims.

Given his claims, the Lalonde Report outlined a strategy for reducing health care costs "by empowering everyone in the community to identify their health agenda, and to develop agencies by which these could be 'advocated' at the neighborhood level, and then mediated by open access to government agencies."[19] The idea was that the government would not just provide health services but would also offer "the Canadian people protection, information and services through which they themselves become partners with health professionals in the preservation and enhancement of their vitality."[20] In effect, the Lalonde Report laid out a strategy for transferring much of the responsibility for health and well-being to individuals and local communities. Lalonde's goal was to incite the moderation of "insidious habits" and environmental risks while at the same time pushing for greater knowledge of human biology: "The Government of Canada now intends to give to human biology, the environment and lifestyle as much attention as it has to financing of the health care organizations so that all four avenues to improved health are pursued with equal vigor. Its goal will be not only to add years to our life but life to our years, so that all can enjoy the opportunities offered by increased economic and social justice."[21] He outlined four avenues for addressing population health: human biology, lifestyles, environment, and the health care system. These four areas made up the core of his conceptual framework, what he called the Health Field Concept.

His Health Field Concept was meant as a tool with which to analyze, determine, and respond to the health needs of Canadians. In other words, both the problems and the solutions to health were sought in one of the four avenues he outlined. Yet, since Lalonde had already determined that the health care system was neither the cause of nor the answer to the self-imposed and environmental risks Canadians confronted, this led to a more intensive focus on the first three. Further, since environmental risks are defined as being linked to human activity—although as he points out they are beyond the control of any one individual—the unstated conclusion of his analysis is that it is either human biology or behavior that is to blame for causing the death or illness of the Canadian population; thus one or both of these factors must be changed to prevent such a fate. His main point, then, is that people were free to "choose their own poison," but they were also increasingly obligated to choose wisely and in such a way as to create the least negative repercussions for fellow citizens, so that "all can enjoy the opportunities offered by increased economic and social justice."[22] To put it another way, Canadians were encouraged to exercise a regulated freedom.

Together, the Declaration of Alma Ata, the Lalonde Report, and the Ottawa Charter have informed the predominant global thinking on health promotion for the last five decades. The Alma Ata and Ottawa conferences provided important forums for this thinking to emerge and be debated assembling diverse actors and agendas in order to develop a global health agenda that could be utilized in diverse contexts and on behalf of the poorest and least resourced populations. In other words, they set the tone for what was to become a primary component of the global development agenda. The Lalonde Report established norms for how developed nations could go about addressing the increase in chronic and "self-induced" health problems and the coincident rising costs of health care.

From Health for All to Healthy People

The approach adopted in Canada has been reflected in that of other developed countries, such as the United Kingdom and the United States. Indeed, its influence was evident in the first surgeon general's report, *Healthy People: The Surgeon General's Report on Health Promotion and Disease Prevention*, produced by the U.S. Department of Health, Education, and Welfare in 1979. As stated in the foreword to the report, its purpose was to encourage a second public health revolution in the history of the United States, the first being that fought against infectious diseases, which spanned the 19th and the first half of the 20th centuries. The report, which strongly echoed the Lalonde Report in Canada, names the main causes of death in the United States: cardiovascular disease, cancer, and accidents. The causes of these "modern killers," as outlined by then secretary of health, education and welfare, Joseph A. Califano, in his introductory comments to the report, are summarized as follows:

> We are killing ourselves by our own careless habits
>
> We are killing ourselves by carelessly polluting the environment
>
> We are killing ourselves by permitting harmful social conditions to exist—conditions like poverty, hunger and ignorance—which destroy health, especially for infants and children.[23]

The idea that individuals are responsible for their own illness and death is clear in these comments. The creation of the Office of Disease Prevention and Health Promotion in 1976 and the subsequent publication of this report had a strong impact on the direction of national public health services in the United States. As laid out in follow-up documents, *Healthy People 2000* and *Healthy People 2010*, health promotion has become one of the primary strategies for the national health agenda as defined by the U.S. Department of Health and Human Services. The National Institutes of Health, the National Academy of Medicine, the Centers for Disease Control and Prevention, and the Office of Minority Health and the Office on Women's Health in the U.S. Department of Health and Human Services, among others, subsequently jumped on the health promotion bandwagon, providing funding for and conducting research on health promotion programs especially for poor and minority populations who were perceived as placing an undue and unwanted burden on everyone else.

This focus is highlighted in the preface to *Healthy People 2000*, which states that "the problems of particularly difficult target groups, such as those living at the extremities of life as measured by age or circumstance, are being measured because of their special significance to, and impact upon, all of us."[24] Foundations and nonprofits across the United States have also consequently made health promotion a central component of their funding and service delivery strategies. The March of Dimes, the Kresge Foundation, and the California Endowment, to name just a few, have all provided funding for health promotion programs meant to address health issues of concern to low-income, minority, and immigrant communities. The Robert Wood Johnson Foundation has been at the forefront of promoting a national "culture of health."

Primary Health Care for Global Equality

In the final analysis, creating a healthier social order will depend on reaching across traditional barriers and replacing global pillage with a global village—where everyone's basic needs are equitably and flexibly met.[25]

From the outset, health promotion was conceived as a strategy for giving communities more of a say and more responsibility in the care they receive. Participation was conceived not only as a right to be exercised by those most affected, but also as a duty for them to take some action on their own behalf. As stated in the Declaration of Alma Ata, the primary health care strategy "*requires* and promotes maximum community and individual *self-reliance* and participation in the planning, organization, operation and control of primary health care."[26] Although that Declaration does call for individuals and communities to play a more active role in their health care, the original intention of this transfer of responsibility was understood as providing more voice and power to rural communities all over the world who previously had little access to health care and little say in what services they did receive. In other words, it was meant to respond to the idea that health care is a human right that should involve and be exercised by those humans whose health is in question and not based on technical or political solutions formulated from the top down.

This social democratic focus informed the content and the political agenda of the Declaration of Alma Ata. Indeed, the decision to adopt primary health care as a global health promotion strategy was debated and unanimously agreed to at the Alma Ata Conference not only because it provided a cost-effective, intersectoral approach to health, but also because it involved the most affected individuals and communities.[27] This horizontal approach was in sharp contrast to the medical model practiced in the 1950s, mainly by the WHO and the United States, which were criticized for being too vertical.

The focus on health care as a right reflects a strong concern with social justice in the formative years of the global health promotion agenda, one meant to redress economic and political inequality between the global south and north. The move toward listening to the most marginalized populations in the global south was part of a growing global trend that criticized modernization models used to "develop" the global south and sought to replace them with more appropriate and sensitive development models. Part of the reason that the Alma Ata Conference was focused on establishing primary health care services in "developing" countries was informed by the spread of nationalist, anti-imperialist, and leftist movements in many of the "less developed" countries, as a result of the newly won independence of former colonial states, and in light of a 1974 resolution passed by the UN General Assembly on the establishment of a New International Economic Order, conceptualized as a way to uplift "less developed" countries.[28] The conference participants at Alma Ata responded to the U.N. resolution and its political precursors adding these words to the Declaration: "The International Conference on Primary Health Care calls for urgent and effective national and international action to develop and implement primary health care throughout the world and particularly in developing countries in a spirit of technical cooperation and in keeping with a New International Economic Order."[29]

As evidenced in the WHO-UNICEF joint report, by the time of the Alma Ata conference, many of the countries in the global south had already taken matters into their own hands and successfully initiated their own model health programs to deliver a basic but comprehensive program of primary health care services covering poor, rural populations. It was from these programs that the conference participants took the name "primary health care," as well as some of the primary methods for promoting health in rural areas.[30] As cited earlier, one of the countries that had begun to address the primary health care needs of its population prior to Alma Ata was communist China. Part of their national strategy incorporated the use of community health care workers (community health workers), or "barefoot doctors," who were trained in basic health care and whose efforts, which included a mix of "traditional" and allopathic medicine, were dedicated especially to rural, agricultural regions. Mao's plan to turn peasants into barefoot doctors was implemented in 1956 as part of the "Great Leap Forward," intended to increase agricultural production by ensuring a healthy workforce, and which gained visibility with the entrance of the People's Republic of China into the United Nations system in 1971.[31] Part of this platform was a backlash against Western style "elite" medicine and its "bourgeois" policies, as "self-interested" physicians, who only treated rare and difficult diseases rather than addressing the common parasites plaguing the Chinese peasantry, were denounced as "disregarding the masses."[32] Accordingly, this national model was based on preventive rather than curative services.

The success of the rural "barefoot doctors" partly lay in the fact that they served the communities from which they came. Another factor that played into their success had to do with what Sidel and Sidel have called the Chinese focus on individuality, but not individualism.[33] That is, the national health care strategy was based on the idea that individuals should cultivate their unique talents not for the sake of individual development and fulfillment, but for the good of the larger society.[34] Public health education campaigns and the work of community health workers in China were based on this ethic of responsibility to the larger social body.

In the 1960s, the Christian Medical Commission, a specialized organization of the World Council of Churches and the Lutheran World Federation whose members worked in the global south, also trained village health workers at the grassroots level to use simple methods and essential drugs.[35] Several of its programs, including the village health worker model, were already known to WHO staff members when a formal collaboration was established between the World Health Organization and the Christian Medical Commission in 1974. At Alma Ata, the use of community health workers, based on the Chinese and Christian Medical Commission models, was emphasized as one of the cornerstones of comprehensive health care.[36]

From Comprehensive Primary Health Care to Selective Primary Health Care

Despite the existence of successful models in the developing world and the political will of international health organizations such as WHO and UNICEF for achieving global social and economic equality through the implementation of a primary health care agenda, a report that emerged on the heels of Alma Ata would change the shape, direction, and politics of health promotion. This document entitled "Selective Primary Health Care: An Interim Strategy for Disease Prevention in Developing Countries," was authored by Julia Walsh and Kenneth S. Warren, both researchers then working for the Rockefeller Foundation in the United States. The goal of their paper was to outline an "interim" strategy or entry point through which the primary health care agenda could be achieved.[37] While the paper itself did not criticize the Alma Ata Declaration, it was a response to criticism that the goals outlined in Alma Ata were too broad and, therefore, unachievable. Consequently, the report proposed "selective" primary health care, which included a package of low-cost technical interventions to tackle the main disease problems of poor countries. It also emphasized attainable goals and cost-effective planning.

At first the recommendations in the paper were broad and unclear, focusing primarily on the diseases of infants, such as diarrhea, and those occurring due to lack of immunization. Over time, however, they were reduced to four primary areas: growth monitoring, oral rehydration techniques, breastfeeding, and immunization, which came to be known as GOBI.[38] As Marcos Cueto explains, these four were chosen not only because they were necessary and important for keeping children healthy and alive but also because they were easy to monitor and evaluate as they were measurable and offered clear targets.[39] This meant that "funding would be easier to obtain because indicators of success and reporting could be produced more rapidly."[40] Some agencies went on to add food supplementation, female literacy, and family planning to their GOBI agendas. Other diseases and illnesses, such as acute respiratory illness, were not added, however, despite their prevalence in poor countries, because "they were thought to require the administration of antibiotics that non-medical practitioners in many of the affected countries were not allowed to use."[41] Importantly, addressing the social and economic conditions affecting infant and child health status were also not included as part of the "selective" primary health care strategy.

As the foregoing suggests, a shift in thinking occurred, in which funding imperatives rather than comprehensive health outcomes became the priority driving the health promotion agenda. This shift was accompanied by a change in perspective regarding the goal of health promotion, wherein health became conceptualized as an end to be achieved through goals and objectives measurable by the biology of program participants rather than as a means for achieving the more abstract political goals conceptualized at Alma Ata, such as social justice and equality. This shift was further consolidated at a 1979 conference sponsored by the Rockefeller Foundation at their conference center in Bellagio, Italy. The conference, entitled "Health and Population in Development," was attended by representatives of many influential U.S. institutions, including Robert S. McNamara, former secretary of defense and then president of the World Bank; Maurice Strong, chairman of the Canadian International Development and Research Center; David Bell, vice president of the Ford Foundation; and John J. Gillian, administrator of the U.S. Agency for International Development.[42]

At the meeting, McNamara advocated business management methods and clear sets of goals for achieving poverty reduction, a line of thinking that resonated with the "selective" approach to primary care outlined by the Rockefeller scholars. The fact that governments and health agencies could demonstrate a return on financial investment through targeted, short-term strategies helped to legitimate the monies they had already received and to secure additional funding for their programs. It also bolstered the case for selective, rather than comprehensive, primary health care as an effective health strategy, despite evidence that comprehensive health care was working in "developing" countries. Given the need to show "measurable results," as outlined in the Rockefeller report and at the Bellagio conference, those diseases and illnesses that could not be easily or quickly dealt with were left outside the selective primary health care agenda.

This shift in thinking sparked a debate between those who favored a selective approach to primary health care and those who advocated the more holistic view, as outlined at Alma Ata, a debate that turned on two different approaches to health and development. On the one hand, the leaders of UNICEF, the World Bank, the Rockefeller Foundation and, eventually, the Pan American Health Organization, as well as medical doctors who were averse to moving to rural communities where their salaries and living conditions would not be commensurate with their education level or adequately remunerate the cost of their studies, advocated technological solutions to what these actors considered the "natural" reality of high mortality rates caused by illness and disease in poor countries. Their solutions were embodied in the GOBI agenda, which measured the height and weight of children, provided oral rehydration solution, taught mothers the importance of breastfeeding (in spite of the aggressive global campaign by Nestlé and other corporations to undermine this effort and sell baby formula), and implemented immunization campaigns.

On the other hand, the leaders of WHO and critical scholars in the global south challenged this technocratic approach, advocating a political solution to disease, which they perceived was a socially and economically driven problem coming from the global north. These critics called the distribution of oral rehydration solution a Band-Aid in areas where clean water and sanitation were the real issues. They charged that selective primary health care was a destructive "counter-revolution" that attracted professionals, funding agencies, and governments looking for short-term goals.[43] Because selective primary health care instantiated a policy of categorical interventions or a disease-by-disease approach to health, it was accused of weakening public health infrastructures by redirecting funds away from campaigns addressing the social determinants of health, thereby working contrary to an environmental approach to health promotion.[44] According to Hall and Taylor, the move to selective primary health care had the following effect: "[It] took the decision-making power away from the communities and delivered it to foreign consultants with technical expertise in . . . specific areas. These technical experts, often employed by the funding agencies, were subject to the policies of their agencies, not the communities. Selective primary health care reintroduced vertical programs at the cost of comprehensive primary health care."[45]

The context in which this debate ensued was largely informed by the emergence of neoliberalism as the new economic global model and the turbulence of inflation, recession, foreign debt, and structural adjustment policies affecting developing countries during the 1980s. As a result, budgets for health funding were cut in both the global north and the global south, and, consequently, selective primary health care gained salience while transferring responsibility for securing population health to individuals and the market, and away from governments. Within neoliberal rationality, selective primary health care represented what was perceived to be an acceptable balance between scarcity and choice. *Whose* choice, however, is the question. While developed countries voluntarily implemented neoliberal health care following the new government policies of the United States and England, developing countries were forced into this approach as part of structural adjustment packages funded by global financial institutions like the International Monetary Fund and the World Bank.[46] Given the north–south imbalance in economic power, and the turbulence of economic instability in the global south, the agendas of the global north consequently trickled into the south through international humanitarian and philanthropic organizations.

A Neoliberal Culture of Health

What the documents and conferences discussed thus far in the chapter bring together at a global level extends beyond just a focus on primary health care. They also bring to bear a rationality for rule or *mentality* that seeks to transform the subjectivities of target populations in accordance with political objectives produced at the international and national levels. For example, primary health care is a means for holding individuals and communities responsible and accountable for their health. Although this is evident in all of the documents, the Lalonde Report makes it clear that health and lifestyle "choices" are connected, and people with "insidious habits" are not only accountable to themselves but are an economic and social drain on the entire nation. Given this, entire communities and, indeed, nations, are called upon to help keep those with unhealthy behaviors in check. This is apparent in the idea forwarded in the U.S. surgeon general's report that "the problems of particularly difficult target groups . . . have significance to, and impact upon, all of us." Extended to the global south, we see that the physical state and the lifestyle "choices" of the impoverished are a problem not only for the countries within which they reside but also for industrialized nations whose economic and political security is both tied to and dependent upon the health status of poorer nations and poorer people.

Additionally, the imperative of health as an economic development strategy is embedded in a growing health promotion complex that has taken on global dimensions, bringing together actors, institutions, and ideas engaged in addressing the global problems of health, development, and security. This complex relies on strong communication and connection between actors, from policy papers circulated in international health venues to the provision of health education at the local level, as proposed by Lalonde. More recently, this complex relies on the connection of the health of all actors to the market, whether directly through their lifestyle and consumption practices or indirectly through their nation's role as an economic player in the global market. One of the unstated goals of the health promotion complex is the social and economic development of countries in the global south, so they can become important economic and political partners for those in the global north. Further, industrialization is promoted through these documents as a means for ensuring peace and safety. Given this, not only are various actors assembled in the imperative to health but so are various political, economic, and social agendas that respond to the needs and desires of those in the global north. This assemblage demonstrates how global health problems are defined and toward what end. The culture of health being promoted through this health promotion complex is also a culture of neoliberal capitalism.

A corollary to the foregoing point is that the global health promotion agenda is invested in producing "modern" subjects by building their human capital. Indeed, nations are only as strong and capable as their citizens. Several of the components that make up a modern subject include understanding oneself as an individual; a will to the domination of nature, especially one's own; the knowledge and use of science and technology; and a will to rationality and truth. Within the very definition of health promotion outlined in the Ottawa Charter, we see that the imperative to health is also an imperative to become modern: "The process of enabling people to *increase control over*, and to improve their health . . . to reach a state of complete, physical, mental, and social well-being, an individual or group must be able to identify and realize aspirations, to satisfy needs, and *to change or cope with the environment*. People cannot achieve their fullest health potential unless they are able to *take control* of those things which determine their health."[47] Here, the understanding of one's "self" as an individual who not only can but should aspire to control her nature is evident. This is a secular perspective that posits the individual as the ultimate guarantor of and authority on her existence. The formula for her to achieve this control is through control of those environmental and social aspects that have an impact on her health, thereby extending her will to domination beyond herself to the people and things around her. Some of the methods to take control, and the objects to be controlled, are reflected in the guidelines for achieving health for all. These include achieving the proper body weight for children, access to clean water and trained birth attendants, adequate sanitary facilities, and child care. Other methods are reflected in the Lalonde Report, which prescribes a reduction in bad habits through "proper" health education and behavior modification. The achievement of these things necessitates the knowledge and use of science and technology, either by individuals themselves or by a health "expert," in order to "empower" people and build their capacity for self-control and self-government.

The articulation and achievement of the health for all goals demonstrate a will to rationality and truth—that is, a desire to streamline and control life through the appropriate use of scientific knowledge and technology. The production of epidemiological facts and biostatistics inform this rational endeavor. Health experts with specific scientific and technical knowledge, rather than individuals and communities, outline the problems, the solutions, and the stakes in the imperative to health; individuals and communities are obligated to pursue this imperative through their "duty to be well."[48]

By defining a global health agenda, health experts in international and national arenas are creating rules, definitions, ideas, and, importantly, conceptualizations about human subjects and their "nature," which prescribe the epistemological and ontological forms that people across the globe, and in particular geographic spaces, should adopt in order to preserve and maximize their existence.[49] These forms, although varied, are informed by notions of liberalism. Rose reveals the stakes in this arrangement, explaining that "in becoming so integral to the exercise of political authority, experts gain the capacity to generate 'enclosures,' relatively bounded locales or fields of judgment within which their authority is concentrated, intensified and rendered difficult to countermand."[50] Accordingly, an effect of the scientific truths generated by health promotion experts, conferences, and documents is the development of a "scientific picture" or "regime of representation" that foregrounds what are deemed important or vital political, economic, and social concerns based on a liberal conception of humans and human nature, while backgrounding or subjugating those knowledges, concerns, and representations that do not align with the ideas and agenda of global and national health experts.[51] Indigenous health practices most certainly fall out of this agenda.

As discussed earlier, this scientific picture includes some of the indicators of childhood health and well-being. However, it ignores others either because they must be treated by medical or technical "experts" or, as in the case of the socioeconomic conditions that lead to many of the treatable illnesses, they are harder to deal with given the way the health problems and their solutions are defined. Within this scientific picture, poor and marginalized people (and consequently their belongings and ideas) primarily exist as a lack (unhealthy) or a difference (pathological, abnormal), as not "modern" and thus in need of being modernized (underdeveloped, "developing"), or as without power or capacities and therefore in need of being "empowered" or subjected to "capacity build-ing" activities. In other words, those who are understood to embody a world-view that is not liberal and capitalist must be targeted and transformed in order to fit the picture that has been created about who and what is healthy. They must be educated to change their behavior and to make better health decisions.

The need to more closely and authentically fit the scientific representation of health and accepting the scientific truths that are produced through health and development statistics becomes an ethical imperative that is tied through economic, political, and social domains to the lives of each and all. Given this, it becomes vital for everyone—but especially those in the global south, or those considered to be part of particularly difficult target groups, to learn and embody these scientific truths about health in order to maximize their lives, the lives of those they love, and even the lives of those they don't know but whose geopo-litical or economic destiny is tied to their own.

Through this health politics, health subjects are encouraged to believe that the problems of social and biological existence have technological solutions that can and must be sought in the name of global health, wealth, and security. They are also taught that individuals and communities have an ethical, economic, and political obligation to desire and seek out these technological and scientific solu-tions for themselves through their involvement with experts in primary health care. As the Lalonde Report makes clear, increased morbidity and mortality must be avoided, and life and vitality *must be achieved*. This is the imperative inher-ent in the idea of health for all.

While the foregoing may give the impression that health promotion as a global assemblage has a cohesive structure, I want to show the diversity and complexity of its formation in terms of where it has traveled and who it has sought to engage, as well as the kinds of representations, methods, and forces that it "assembles" in pursuit of its goals. This macro perspective is meant to draw attention to the extensive reach and political power the imperative to health wields, similar in many ways to the strength and breadth of the development apparatus with which it articulates.[52] It is also meant to show how primary health care has political imperatives beyond just making people healthy. It is both a tool for social justice and a way to promote neoliberal citizenship, both of which promise empowerment.

I now turn to a brief discussion of how the primary health care agenda was adopted and has evolved in Mexico. Because La Agencia modeled its health promotion program on the Mexican model, it is important to understand how it operates, with what other agendas it articulates, and what rationalities inform its implementation. As with the global primary health care agenda, the Mexican primary health care model is also linked to an antipoverty agenda, and has reconfigured its methods under neoliberalism. The "culture of health" that it promotes has therefore been consistent with neoliberal values.

Mexico: Health Promotion as a Poverty Reduction Strategy

In 1974, the Mexican Institute of Social Security (Instituto Mexicano del Seguro Social-IMSS) implemented a program to extend primary health care services throughout the nation, especially to the marginalized rural populations. The program was entitled Mexico's National Program of Social Solidarity for Community Cooperation (Programa Nacional de Solidaridad Social por Cooperación Communitaria). It was developed based on a 1973 modification of the social security law, which sought to address the extreme poverty and profound marginalization of the population, whose capacity to contribute to the social security system was limited. Three years later, the Mexican government would create the General Coordination of the National Plan for Depressed Zones and Marginalized Groups (Coordinación General del Plan Nacional de Zonas Deprimidas y Grupos Marginados-Coplamar) as an additional strategy for combating poverty. In 1977 these two programs were joined with the goal of extending health services throughout Mexico.

In 1983, and based on the recommendations developed at Alma Ata, IMSS-Coplamar implemented a model of integrated health care based on the concept of primary health care. Similar to the ideas discussed at Alma Ata, the model called for community participation in solving local health problems. Community involvement was achieved through the institutionalization of a general assembly, a health committee, and a group of volunteer health promoters at the local levels. In addition, the model called for coverage by one physician (usually a fifth-year medical student called a *pasante*, a term that can be loosely translated as someone who is "passing through") and one nurse's aide who would spend part of their time in a rural health unit or hospital. Volunteer rural health assistants would also be trained for communities lacking a permanent facility. Although the clinical services provided were free of charge, local community members were expected to donate up to ten days of their labor to construct and maintain the clinic.[53] In exchange, the health teams would provide basic pharmaceuticals, general outpatient consultations, mother–infant care and family planning, health education, nutritional information, sanitation promotion, immunizations, and control of communicable diseases.[54]

This early iteration of the primary health care program in Mexico reflects what Rose has identified as liberalism's concern with social welfare. He explains that under this form of governance, "the State was to take responsibility for generating an array of technologies of government that would 'social-ize' both individual citizenship and economic life in the name of collective security."[55] As Rose describes it, "This was a formula of rule somewhere between classical liberalism and nascent socialism."[56] Certainly this socialized citizenship is evident in the IMSS-Coplamar program, which required the "voluntary" participation of community residents in the building and maintenance of their clinic. It is also present in the idea that by utilizing those health care services, which they have paid for with their labor, community residents will be contributing to the economic and health security of the collective body (variously defined as the local community and the larger Mexican nation). Finally, the resemblances to a socialist model of health care become evident when one considers that these programs were centrally planned and funded by the federal government in Mexico City, although they were implemented at the local level and under the guise of the "voluntary" individual participation of the promotoras, health committee members, rural assistants, and laborers. Significantly, this voluntary model of community participation closely resembles the system of *tequio*, or communal labor, which is still practiced in many indigenous Mexican communities today and which is one of the bases for claims to autonomous indigenous governance.

In the wake of the debt crisis in the early 1980s and under the guidance of the World Bank, Mexico undertook the implementation of structural adjustment programs. These programs, following the broader health promotion agenda, laid out a strategy whereby targeted methods and objectives for achieving economic stability could be achieved. One method was to increasingly decentralize government health services to individual states. Decentralization led to decreased social spending and a deterioration of health care services in the most impoverished Mexican states.[57] In a seeming paradox, these changes were undertaken

in the same year that Mexico integrated the right to health into article 4 of its
Constitution. This is only a paradox, however, if one assumes that the Mexican
government was going to provide the health services. Indeed, decentralization
pushed responsibility for health care provision onto the states, and the states,
in turn, made health care the responsibility of individuals and community members. The role of the government was to make available the means (technical
assistance, program curricula, etc.) for individuals and communities to take care
of themselves.

Given this, it is not surprising that one year later, in accordance with the
General Health Law (La Ley General de Salud), it was announced that community participation was both a responsibility and an obligation of people and
institutions. In what form the community could actually participate in the
targeted and decentralized programs conceptualized by the logic of structural
adjustment was narrowly defined. As Laurell argues in reference to these changes,
"It becomes clear that decentralization, at best, means that local authorities or
community groups can select one or more programs from a pre-established menu
and participation means that those involved should contribute resources to the
program, be they fiscal, economic or human, or, alternatively, they should adopt
prescribed behaviors."[58] She goes on to denounce the "cost-efficiency strategy of
poverty programs" utilized by international financial institutions to achieve their
goals in Latin America as "a technical device derived from management logic."
Citing DALYs (disability adjusted life years) for health actions used by the World
Bank, and "Social Gaps" utilized by the Inter-American Development Bank for
calculating cost-efficiency, Laurell argues that these approaches suffer from "serious conceptual limitations" insofar as they extract simple causal relations from
complex processes, and also because "these techniques are frequently used to
justify service restrictions and turn social priorities into a purely numerical matter
that is alien to values and ethics."[59]

Although Laurell sees these strategies as void of ethical content, ethics is
precisely what they are concerned with—the ethics of the program recipients,
that is. This concern was consolidated by the 1985 announcement that individual and community participation was to be a permanent component of Mexico's development plans for modernization.[60] The link between community
participation and modernization was outlined in the 1990 World Bank's *World
Development Report: Poverty*, which offered a two-part strategy for attacking
poverty, including labor intensive growth and investment in the human capital
development of the poor.[61] The latter, which was concerned with health and
education, posited the creation of active citizens who could engage in the market and therefore manage their own well-being and security.[62] The direction

subsequently followed by the Mexican government reflects the influence of this World Bank report and demonstrates Laurell's critique that program options for community participation in their health care were increasingly constrained under neoliberalism.

In 1997, a new antipoverty program, named Progresa (Program of Education, Health and Nutrition 1997–2000), was created under the administration of Ernesto Zedillo. The program was renamed Oportunidades (Program for Human Development Opportunities) under President Vicente Fox (2000–2006). This program operated by providing the poorest Mexican families with cash transfers for their families' nutritional and educational needs on condition that mothers and their children abide by the program requirements.[63] In exchange for a minimal cash incentive, female heads of household, who were the designated beneficiaries of the program, were required to fulfill a series of requirements, including attending monthly health workshops, ensuring that their family members attend medical appointments, and overseeing their children's school attendance.

In addition, mothers were obligated to ensure that their adolescent children attend an after-school program focused on teen health issues (primarily addressing reproductive health and sexuality). As part of the program, mothers were given the cash incentive, and they were also taught how to open a bank account, save their money, and invest in good nutrition for their families. At the same time, their children were taught how to invest in themselves by learning the value of an education for their own future and that of their parents. Because the program works from the premise that the cash transfers will provide incentives for the impoverished to invest in their own health and education, it is commonly referred to as a "social investment" program.

In addition to the empowerment activities for mothers and children, the Oportunidades program also had a disciplinary component. In order to oversee women's participation, a committee of community promotion acted as a liaison between female beneficiaries and the government. Further, a doctor and social worker were assigned to work with families in order to document their progress in obtaining the program's objectives. As in the previous models, a number of promotoras (the number depends on how many beneficiaries there are in the community) were also designated to oversee a number of families (usually ten to fifteen) who they must visit periodically for a period of up to three years. In their home visits, the promotoras checked to see that the water for household use was boiled, that there was no standing water outside, and that the trash was burned, and they tried to detect any health symptoms or conditions, among other things, that family members were experiencing. When a health condition, such as pregnancy, was detected, the promotora was charged with reporting it to the local medical assistant or doctor for follow-up. The health surveillance role of the promotora in the Oportunidades program was vital for collecting epidemiological information on the geographic area covered by the local hospital.[64]

Managing Future Risks

The key objective of cash transfer programs is to change the behavior of the poor to allow them to manage risk better while increasing the possibilities for their children to successfully and productively participate in the labor market in the future. As Lucy Lucissano explains, conditionality and managing future risks are tied together to promote security through increased earning power in the future.[65] Although the program's primary architect, Santiago Levy, conceptualized the program as providing equal opportunity to all Mexicans by taking advantage of their right to health and education, more critical assessments of the program have called attention to the ways that Oportunidades turns rights into responsibilities by obligating women to fulfill the program requirements or else lose their cash transfer.[66] By turning women into market citizens while turning the lives and activities of their children into an economic investment in the future, the conditional cash transfer strategy exhibits aspects of both liberal and neoliberal governmentalities. As Rose explains, under liberal welfarism the family was to be instrumentalized as a *social machine*—both *made* social and utilized to create sociality—implanting the techniques of responsible citizenship under the tutelage of experts and in relation to a variety of sanctions and rewards.[67]

As with IMSS-Coplamar, Oportunidades attempted this socialization by turning a program for social protection and social education into a way for beneficiaries to fulfill their social obligation and social responsibility to the collective health and security of the community and the nation. The rewards beneficiaries received, however, were also what linked their citizenship practices to the market. Rose is again instructive. He writes, "Monetarization plays a key role in breaching welfare enclosures within the networks of social government. Transforming activities—operating on a patient, educating a student, providing a social work interview for a client—into cash terms establishes new relations of power."[68] Under Oportunidades, the cash terms utilized to produce social citizenship reconfigure the terms of "community participation" as they were established under IMSS-Coplamar. Now, rather than paying with their "voluntary" labor to be healed, program beneficiaries are also paid to stay healthy and educated. The minimal stipend they received was not enough for them to pay for any substantial expenses, however, but it was enough to incite their participation in the market and increase the monetarization of their lives and health.

The social investment programs have led to the increased economization of society, especially those who have been outside or on the periphery of the market, while at the same time exposing the poor and marginalized to neoliberal governance. In addition, by targeting recipients based on ethnicity, these programs served as a strategy to quell indigenous protest against the government at a time when indigenous groups were beginning to organize and demand rights and recognition.[69] Because these programs were implemented only in communities that had the infrastructure to operationalize them, they had the added effect of excluding some of the most impoverished communities, thereby creating resentments between those perceived as being the haves and those who were the have-nots.[70] They, therefore, shielded the government from indigenous backlash while at the same time further dividing indigenous communities.

The goal of Oportunidades has been to achieve the autonomous and healthy development of the socially and economically disadvantaged who were living in conditions of marginality by fostering their active participation in their health and well-being. If successful, the program would alleviate the undue burden that the poor and disadvantaged were seen to impose on society. Unfortunately, although poor women and their children accumulate human capital, in rural areas where wage labor is scarce, they have limited or no venues for cashing in on their investments. For this reason, Lucissano is skeptical of the program's ability to achieve its goals due to the instability of the Mexican economy, the precariousness of work, and high levels of poverty and inequality in Mexico.[71] In other words, she is skeptical precisely because of the persistence of those conditions that these social investment programs were meant to alleviate. To the extent that these structural conditions remain unchanged, so, too, does the health of those who participate in the opportunities offered by these programs

Given the influence of international financial institutions in shaping social policy in Latin America, the "Mexican model" for poverty reduction has been adopted in other parts of Latin America, such as Brazil, Chile, Ecuador, Nicaragua, Panamá, Paraguay, and El Salvador. Conditional cash transfers have also been tested in New York City as an antipoverty strategy and they have been adopted in other countries, such as Brazil, Canada, and South Africa, among others.[72]

Health Promotion as an Anti-Politics Machine

The shift in the direction of primary health care represents a move away from the social democratic postwar ideals that informed the development of the Declaration of Alma Ata to a neoliberal global agenda in which individualism, free market, deregulation, and decentralization become hegemonic.[73] Within this new economic scheme, health care was increasingly privatized, as the market was "seen as the perfect mechanism for assuring the life of the population—for averting the risks linked to old age, ill health, poverty, accidents, and so forth."[74] A consequence of market-based health care is that many people who need drugs do not have access to them because they cannot afford to buy them. Furthermore, in many regions, the implementation of selective primary health care has simply become an extension of pre-existing medical services, in which selective primary health care provides a first point of contact for rural communities who can then be incorporated into the medical establishment, rather than prevented from becoming dependent on doctors, hospitals, and other health workers as was initially envisioned at Alma Ata.

In light of this vertical, categorical, and market-based approach to health care, certain diseases are prevented from inclusion in the selective primary health care agenda, and essential drugs also become difficult or impossible to obtain because they are too expensive. Trade agreements, such as the Trade-Related Intellectual Property Rights, further complicated the situation by monopolizing access to essential medication as well as to the knowledge used to produce the medication.[75] This dynamic sets up a paradox in which rural clinics, which lack medicines, technology, and doctors, cannot help those that have been encouraged by selective primary health care programs to access them. This paradox is further extended when one analyzes the conditional cash transfer strategy that builds the human capital of poor populations but provides them no employment opportunities to utilize their skills and knowledge.

The move to selective primary health care represents a return to primary *medical* care, wherein medical and technological solutions guided by neoliberal economic methodologies and focused on achieving quantifiable biological goals are given precedence over the proposed political solutions that address the socioeconomic factors leading to unequal morbidity and mortality rates in the global south and among the poor in the global north. Although the neoliberal economic climate clearly did not favor the implementation of comprehensive primary health care, critical scholars link its demise to the political agendas of those in the global north. Hall and Taylor suggest that "politicians and aid experts from developed countries could not accept the core primary health care principles that communities in developing countries would have responsibility for planning and implementing their own healthcare services."[76] Indeed, "if the goals [of the Ottawa Charter] were to be obtained, it would require drastic changes in power relations both at the global and the national level."[77] Drastic changes did occur, but they were not necessarily the changes envisaged at Alma Ata. As Thomas and Weber explain,

> Whereas the achievement of health as a human right as envisaged at Alma Ata required health to be seen as a public good, the neoliberal development orthodoxy of the 1980s and early 1990s interpreted it instead in terms of its privatization potential. The overarching neoliberal development strategy—based on the promotion of economic growth through structural adjustment of national economies and the liberalization of trade, investment and finance—was to provide the context for the development of global and national health care policies. The new economic orthodoxy that envisaged the comprehensive withdrawal of state influence in markets had the effect of crowding out any political momentum created for cooperative approaches that included redistributive provisions.[78]

In this new political-economic climate, participation, empowerment, and the imperative to health also took on new dimensions. Health had been conceived as the duty and social responsibility of the world community since Alma Ata, a conception of health that was couched in a social democratic rationality that sought social and economic equality between and among the members of the global community. Within this conception, population health and welfare were seen as something in which governments had a strong role to play through provision of methods, agendas, and ideas that could help communities and societies exercise their right to health care and their duty to be well. The responsibility of the population was conceived of as complementary to the role of government, and empowerment was understood as fostering civic participation and a deeper understanding of those socioeconomic and political conditions that bear on health.[79]

In the neoliberal context, by contrast, the collective and social aspects of primary health care concerned with equality of outcome were replaced with a focus on equality of inputs, or what has come to be known as equality of opportunity. One of the primary "inputs" to be manipulated in this rationality is the physical body as the site of health. Thus, individuals are called upon to build their knowledge and capacities for "self"-care while "equality of opportunity" is redefined as equal access to the market. Health education focuses on the technical and biomedical information that will effectively and efficiently achieve the target goals of governments, funding agencies, and international health organizations advocating strategies such as GOBI. This includes an increased focus on access and use of clinical care as a prevention strategy, accompanied by increased reliance on health "experts" and medical professionals at the international and national, rather than local, levels. Meanwhile the economic and technical aspects of global, national, and individual health are emphasized. Although still couched in terms of social well-being as opposed to individual health, concepts such as social *investment* and social *capital* that have been utilized to justify and fortify the global health promotion complex, reveal a socioeconomic perspective of humans and their activities and illuminate the kinds of capitalist cultural imperatives at work.

Through targeted marketing interventions meant to educate and build capacities for health, people are provided the opportunity to make responsible choices in terms of the ways they invest their time and energy so that, like the international agencies designing and funding health promotion programs, they can reap the most return on their investments. Those individuals whose capacities or education are seen as deficient for exercising the opportunities available to them are often identified by funders and governments for more intensive or longer-term health education and capacity-building activities. In the global south these have become known as "social investment programs," and they are linked to government-run antipoverty or human development strategies that require beneficiaries and their families to participate in targeted health and education activities. This is the strategy at the heart of conditional cash transfer schemes like Oportunidades. In the global north, education and capacity-building activities often include health education workshops, health literacy programs, and other health promotion activities that are also targeted, and whose goal is often to increase access to medical care and to change individual behavior. These programs are paid for by both public and private funds.

Such neoliberal interventions, directed at maximizing the health and vitality of human bodies within a prescribed behavioral framework, demonstrate the ways in which the reconfiguration of political and ethical selves also becomes a goal of targeted health promotion efforts. Because this reconfiguration is meant to occur according to the established goals and objectives of health promotion programs, the social democratic aspects of the process are circumscribed, and the political role of agenda-setting is obscured. As we saw in the GOBI agenda, not only are parents encouraged to monitor the growth of their children, they are also encouraged to learn what is "normal" height and weight according to a child's age and, more importantly, to desire and value having their child attain that normal measurement.

The goal of growth, the measurements for establishing "normal" growth, and the participation of parents in monitoring and surveilling that growth have all been prescribed prior to the arrival of the growth-monitoring program in the community and at the family level. Parental participation is, consequently, narrowly defined. While I am not disparaging the importance of growth monitoring, I do want to highlight how global designs have local implications in terms of what "participation," capacity building, and empowerment entail. In other words, health promotion as conceived by global elites has local implications for health subjectivity. Parents are participating in the health of their children; however, their perceptions, actions, behaviors, beliefs, and desires corresponding to that participation have been influenced by forces and agendas that extend beyond the parent–child interaction.

As a result of including growth monitoring in the selective primary health care agenda, parents, children, individuals, and communities are interpellated into a "truth regime" promoted by the global health promotion complex, and they are encouraged to think about themselves, their families, and life in general in "rational," economic, and technocratic terms. They must calculate the height and weight of their child according to a measurement technology that has been designed and determined by health "experts," according to universal biological "standards" that have been developed in another context. This also means that they must understand and learn about "proper" nutrition, food preparation, and consumption, which, in turn, implies calculating biological life in terms of economic intake (can I afford this food?) with economic output (will my child be productive if I do or don't assure her proper growth?) and monitoring it with economic measures (does my child meet the normal measurements?).

This style of thinking is presented as desirable and positive, especially insofar as it collapses economic well-being with physical health—two predominant factors determining biological survival in a market economy—framing health as a technical problem. Parents who love and care about their children want to embrace this way of thinking and acting because it reassures them that their children are "healthy" (at least as defined within this rationality). Of course, the politics behind the knowledges and methodologies that make this style of reasoning possible are not interrogated. What are interrogated, however, are the bodies of the beneficiaries of the social investment programs, like those I observed while conducting field research in Oaxaca, Mexico, whose monthly measurements, taken by the local doctor with a handheld tape measure and a portable scale, become the marker of success or failure for the program, the government, the international funder, and, not insignificantly, the beneficiary.

The politics trafficked in under an objective-based approach need to be illuminated, especially in light of Ilona Kickbusch's keynote address at a 2006 Healthy People Consortium Meeting in New York. Kickbusch, who was then director of the Division of Health Promotion, Education and Communication at

WHO when she delivered her address, asked, "Does the strategic approach of setting goals and targets really make a difference to population health?" Her answer was, "We do not really know."[80] Although this response might lead us to think that more research is needed to test the success or failure of these targeted strategies before we can know the "truth," James Ferguson's "antipolitics machine" is instructive in deciphering her response. In his studies of development in Lesotho, Ferguson argues that a "failed" program, or one that does not achieve its policy objectives, does not mean that it is a program without consequence. He explains, "It may be that what is most important about a 'development' project is not so much what it fails to do but what it does do; it may be that its real importance in the end lies in [its] 'side effects.'"[81]

Although Kickbusch presents contrasting evidence on the effectiveness of objective- based or targeted approaches in her address, I suggest that, whether or not targeted health promotion programs achieve their intended health outcomes, they are successful in producing political subjects who aspire to embody the "truths" forwarded in the global health promotion complex, whether for economic, social, or biological reasons. I further suggest, as Ferguson found in his research, that policy objectives may have the effect of depoliticizing those very issues they purport to bring to the political agenda. Given this, under neoliberalism, Mexican health promotion programs, like the development apparatus in Lesotho, operate as an "anti-politics machine."

Despite the fact that the opportunities for achieving health are defined within the narrow constraints of program goals, they do not cease to incorporate the entire population as a potential target. Kickbusch and Gleicher make this apparent in their publication on health governance for the twenty-first century: "Public policy can no longer just be delivered. [This] study shows that successful governance for health requires co-production as well as the involvement and cooperation of citizens, consumers and patients. As governance becomes more widely diffused throughout society, working directly with the public can strengthen transparency and accountability."[82] Thus, although the message "health for all" has not changed, a new politics has been ushered in under the old rhetoric, wherein a much-reduced definition of health is complemented by a greatly expanded role for the citizen in ensuring her own health and welfare. This new role is alternatively defined as an opportunity, empowerment, social investment, capacity building, or human development. In sum, it bespeaks a positive and desirable outcome, especially for the poor and marginalized across the globe. Such an outcome easily lends itself to visions of achieving a national "culture of health."

While in many ways the culture of health being promoted appears to resonate with the social democratic goals that informed health promotion's foundation, as mentioned, the ideas, knowledges, rationalities, and technologies it
assembles have changed across time and place. With the shift to "selective" primary health care and under neoliberalism, health promotion has emphasized
certain dimensions, such as individual responsibility and entrepreneurship, and
linked these to the market, while downplaying others, such as the collective
duties and responsibilities communities have by virtue of being in the same
social or geographic milieu. In addition, it has returned to primary medical care
and thus to biomedical, as opposed to social and political, determinants of
health. This means that the "Mexican model of health" is not primarily or even
predominantly Mexican and that, therefore, the values at work in programs that
draw from this model are more informed by neoliberal capitalist agendas and
biomedical imperatives than the local languages, customs, traditions, or cultures
of the people they target.

Conclusion: Empowerment and the Right to Health

In this chapter, I have sought to critically examine the origins of the "Mexican
model of health" by illuminating the travels and translations of the global health
promotion agenda. My objectives have been, first, to show how and why mismatches occur between health program objectives and health program participants and, second, to say that these mismatches are not due to some essentialized
culture or antiscience beliefs of indigenous peoples. Rather, they are due to the
imposition of a set of values, norms, epistemes, and expectations in communities that cannot, by virtue of their social position and structural vulnerability,
always and unconditionally embrace and operationalize them. In order to understand the disjunctures that occur we must pay attention to the cultural politics of health programs, especially to the values, norms, practices, and ethical
principles they operationalize, and to the kinds of health subjects they both assume and attempt to produce, rather than focusing exclusively on the cultures
of program participants.

Just like the populations they target, these programs evolve and change with
the social, political, and economic context. Over time the politics of health
promotion have changed from a more comprehensive model focused on social
justice and equity to a narrowed version driven by economics and technology.
This narrowed version of health promotion became "the flavor of the month"
for empowering vulnerable populations not because it was a culturally competent "Mexican model," but because it was economically salient for international

institutions demanding structural adjustment policies in Mexico. As a result of these demands, the empowerment that neoliberal health promotion promises comes in the form of equal opportunity to market citizenship rather than equal access to life-sustaining health resources and infrastructures. Indeed, such resources were diminished under decentralized health care in Mexico and have been largely relegated in the United States to the domain of health philanthropy. Despite the empowerment rhetoric, then, targeted populations are not participating in setting the health agenda, yet they are still responsible for carrying it out. Thus, political activity by and for the people continues to be at the core of health promotion, even as the community-based promotion of health operates as an "antipolitics machine" dividing communities under neoliberalism.

While community participation is certainly a primary aspect of this new health strategy, health care is now defined as an obligation one owes to oneself, to the larger social body, and to powerful economic actors, as opposed to something governments have a role in providing for the populations they serve. Today, it is as often private funders like Bill Gates as it is governments who set the global health agenda, but private individuals are called to embody the funder's objectives under the guise of exercising their "right" to health. This is what is meant by "empowerment" and "ownership." The idea of ownership that undergirds this model is based on both the literal and a figurative "buy-in" of the health consumer to the values and ideals that health promotion is promoting. This is why the political rationalities carried along in health promotion programs are hegemonic—because they coproduce a lived system of meanings and values that are both constitutive and constituting.

The conjuncture of neoliberalism and biomedicine in the selective primary health care agenda informs the way biological and social problems get defined as technical problems and therefore suggest targeted, technical methods to intervene in these problems. For example, human biology becomes the "problem" for which scientific discourse and technical expertise are the solution. At Alma Ata, "needs" and "help" were defined within a sociopolitical framework focused on human rights and economic development. Subsequently, these have come to be defined within a techno-economic framework characterized by techniques that "are frequently used to justify service restrictions and turn social priorities into a purely numerical matter that is alien from values and ethics."[83] The result is that health and its promotion have come to be thought of as a cost–benefit activity that scales up or down (individual, family, community, region, nation, globe) and that ultimately inheres in the bodies, identities, and cultures of individuals and populations, leaving the political rationalities, cultural practices, epistemic commitments, and economic norms of neoliberal government unexamined.

It turns out, then, that the culture of health being promoted in indigenous communities in California is shaped more by the circulation of neoliberal economic values of individual responsibility and ownership, economic accountability and entrepreneurship, and quantitative measurements than by an abstractly defined Mexican culture. When nonprofits, communities, or even individuals do not or cannot produce the numerical results desired by the funding organization, they risk losing credibility and further support. Health thus functions as a moralizing and economizing technology, teaching people the "right" way to act even as it purports to reflect to them their own cultural, linguistic, and social values. Indeed, culture becomes a tool for transmitting this agenda into diverse populations under the guise of empowerment and self-determination, changing the peoples and practices it targets as it transmits. Thus, the "Mexican model" of health promotion is not so much *reflecting* indigenous culture as *producing* it. Recognizing this dynamic helps explain why there are mismatches between the program participants, who don't readily identify with the information they receive, and the health promoters, who are not so much reflecting to their audience who they are but rather are teaching them who they could and should be as "healthy" neoliberal consumer citizens.

Chapter 4

Números, Números, Números

Making Health Programs Accountable

> **Not everything that can be counted counts,
> and not everything that counts can be
> counted.**

A Culture of Documentation

In the middle of my fieldwork La Agencia moved their main office and changed leadership. Their new office sits on a busy street just outside the downtown of the Central Valley city where I first encountered Ramón, their former executive director. A nondescript storefront adjacent to the freeway and surrounded by concrete, it is easy to miss as you drive by. The beige paneled exterior belies the colorful and lively office within. The interior space is divided into a small waiting room with chairs flanked by end tables covered in informational pamphlets, a large office with several desks and a few shelves, and several smaller offices further in. The large office, visible through the rectangular window that separates the waiting room from the rest of the interior, is decorated with a mix of indigenous artwork, books, plants, and a water cooler. Past the copy machine and down the back hall is a kitchen used for lunch breaks and to prepare food for staff and community events.

As I peruse the pamphlets while waiting for my meeting with Luz, I observe a steady trickle of people coming in, asking questions, and looking for help filling out forms. This is the same dynamic I had seen in another of La Agencia's offices on the Central Coast. Staffed by two *promotoras* (community health workers), Berta who is Triqui and Alicia who is Mixtec, the Central Coast office is a tiny glass-walled structure attached to the back of a bright yellow police station, the word "POLICE" stenciled in bold black letters on the wall above. The space had been donated by the local police chief to help the burgeoning indigenous populations in the region. Resembling a toll booth and lacking a bathroom, which was a huge irritation for both women, but especially Berta who was pregnant at the time, the makeshift Central Coast office, like the one in the Central Valley, served as a hub of activity for the two undocumented indigenous promotoras and the many indigenous migrants they helped.

During my time in the toll booth office, where I sat squeezed between two small desks and a bucket with a mop, I watched scores of indigenous women come in for help, holding crumpled, fingerprint-smudged envelopes with folded papers inside. Trying to figure out which languages and dialects they spoke, the promotoras would eye the forms in the visitors' hands while asking, first in Spanish, *¿En que le puedo ayudar, Señora?* ("How can I help you, Ma'am?"). Surrendering creased envelopes and stacks of papers, the visitors would explain that they needed help dealing with some documentation-related issue. "I need to show my income in order to qualify for food stamps." "My son needs to enroll in school, but I don't know his birthdate and I don't have a birth certificate for him." "They sent me this form but I don't know what to put in the box marked social security." "I need help opening a post-office box to receive my mail." While listening to the visitors, the promotoras would open the envelopes containing phone numbers, street addresses, electricity bills, pay stubs, and other numerical representations of the woman's identity, or that of her loved ones, while simultaneously glancing over the forms to be filled out. *A ver* ("Let's see").

Conventional wisdom in the United States indicates that institutional forms should be written at an eighth-grade level for accessibility. Despite this, many are written at a tenth-grade level.[1] This makes filling out routine forms a significant challenge for most indigenous migrants, especially women. Whether a rental agreement, school enrollment, access to social services, health insurance, or an employment application, every life opportunity for indigenous migrants in the United States requires documentation, and that documentation, in turn, requires basic literacy and numeracy skills. However, many indigenous Mexican migrants have low literacy and numeracy due to having attended school for so few years. For example, on average, indigenous farmworkers in California between the ages of eighteen and twenty-five attended school for six and a half years. Many indigenous females do not make it past the fourth grade, however. By contrast, their mestizo counterparts attend school for a little over seven years.[2]

A huge part of the promotoras' job, then, is to help with reading and writing on behalf of the indigenous community. This can include reading letters from home or translating bills. It can also include writing letters to foundations, as I was asked to do one day when a family came in looking for help. Their little boy, who was a U.S. citizen, had been given hearing aids by a U.S. foundation. The hearing aids, along with the boy's passport, were stolen by the people who his mother, not a U.S. citizen, had entrusted with taking him across the border in Nogales, Texas, while she was being smuggled into the country a bit farther away. At the request of the foundation, the father had to write a letter apologizing for the loss and promising that he would never lose them again.

Unaccustomed to writing formal letters, the promotoras were worried that their written language skills were not strong enough to correspond with a powerful foundation. Consequently, they decided that I should write the letter because, as they explained, I would "know what to say." Angry that the parents had been shamed like this, but cognizant of their need to get new hearing aids for their son, I wrote the letter. In it I acknowledged the generosity of the foundation and the importance of the hearing aids to the child's health. Reflecting the kind of moral responsibility and individual ownership for the loss that was expected by the foundation, I promised that the parents would not lose his hearing aids again. Several weeks after I had written the letter the child received a new set.

Lack of advanced schooling is not the only barrier to filling out forms, however. Indigenous Mexicans are not accustomed to operating within what Luz called "a culture of documentation." As she explained to me, indigenous Oaxacans are not used to continually legitimating their identities, relationships, and personhood by amassing bundles of papers with numbers corresponding to their life activities. Indeed, numerous people affiliated with the indigenous community in California explained to me that indigenous cultures in Oaxaca are oral cultures, which means that the spoken word is as valuable, if not more valuable, than the printed word. Because of the lack of infrastructure in rural communities, indigenous groups have had to rely heavily on the oral transmission of information and on verbal agreements.

This reliance on oral agreements can make them suspicious when they have to sign something they are unable to read. For example, following university research protocol when interviewing human subjects, I asked all interviewees to sign a consent form prior to interviewing them. Rather than fostering increased trust, however, several of my interviewees became more distrustful of me after they had signed. In one case, I interviewed two Triqui women in my apartment where, prior to proceeding, we had a lengthy discussion in Spanish of my research project and their rights in the interview process. They eventually agreed to sign the form. While I directed my questions to both women, only one spoke for both. This was partly due to the other woman not speaking Spanish fluently, but I later learned that it was primarily because she was uncomfortable as a result of signing the consent form. In fact, her friend revealed at the end of the interview that, rather than focusing on answering my questions, she had repeatedly asked her friend in Triqui, "What is that paper for? Why did I sign it?"

The idea that indigenous Oaxacans lack a "culture of documentation" was reinforced when I finally sat down to interview Luz in the Central Valley office. We were discussing immigration reform, but the conversation quickly turned to the importance of documenting everything:

Luz: And another challenge that I think we have yet to see and that I think, unfortunately, is going to be a huge obstacle when they pass migration reform (and we hope that they pass the reform) is that, not only the indigenous but all of us, we don't have the culture of documenting anything. And in the indigenous community especially they have an oral culture. Papers for us are not as important. There [in Mexico] if you give your word, then your word is what is important. You don't have to make a contract and go to the notary to make sure that you fulfill your agreement. Your word is what is important, and it's more valuable. For example, I don't know if you knew this, but the Triquis don't get married with a matrimonial contract. They have a party in which the whole community participates, and certain elders give their permission for the wedding and there is no paper. And this is a problem because when they want to demonstrate that they are married, they don't have a paper, and this is when you have problems with immigration. Because if, for example, they are waiting to get immigration status, then they are going to have to show that they have been here for a certain number of years and that they have been working. But many people throw everything away, or they have unfortunately accepted to work without papers, I mean without a contract and getting paid in cash. So how will the [immigration] agent document their status? And a lot of people say, well, even if it's an electricity bill we will throw it away. Unfortunately, I do this, too! So, here the thing is to learn all of this. It's that you have to learn to document, document, document. Paper, paper for everything, no?

Health Programming and the Audit Culture

If asked, most readers of this book could likely rattle off their Social Security number, telephone number, birth date, street address, and a host of other numbers (including computer passwords, important phone numbers, birth dates of loved ones, the average number of steps recorded on their Fitbit, and so on).

They could also likely produce a number of documents, including birth certificates, driver's licenses, passports, utility bills, and the like to verify that those
numbers correspond to their bodies and identities (brown eyes, brown hair,
150 pounds, size 9 shoe, size 10 pants, and so forth). In the United States we
continually translate our identities into a series of numbers; we affirm our
identities with numbers, and those numbers affirm us.

The paper on which those numbers are written is material proof not only
of our identity but of our existence; it is an extension of ourselves and in some
ways a more valuable and meaningful affirmation of our personhood than the
flesh on our bones. Indeed, the importance of a birth certificate or passport for
verifying not only one's citizenship and relationships but one's very existence
cannot be overstated. To be documented, then, is to have access to a variety of
services. It is a way to claim both political rights and social recognition. By contrast, to lack documentation or to be unaccounted for, even if you are a citizen,
means not only that you will have trouble accessing life-sustaining resources
like health care, but also that you will be suspect and ineligible for personhood
until you can furnish the documentation that proves your identity. As I argued
in chapter 2, to "be" undocumented in the United States is tantamount to being
criminal, a terrorist, subhuman—or, worse, to not existing at all. Cognizant of
this, La Agencia is highly invested in helping both its program participants and
its employees operate within a culture of documentation.

This chapter shows how accounting imperatives, especially those of documentation and quantification, shape the experiences of both the employees and
the program participants in La Agencia's Indigenous Health Project (IHP). An
extension of chapter 3 in which selective or targeted health programming
informed the practices of global health promotion, this chapter demonstrates
how similar imperatives inform programming at a local level through the IHP.
Using the idea of "audit culture," the chapter illustrates the effect that a "culture of documentation" and "rituals of verification" have on health programming in indigenous Mexican migrant communities, particularly as these are
entangled with and influence indigenous cultures, in order to reinforce the point
that there are more cultures at work in the IHP than just those of the populations the programs serve.[3] The entanglements of these various cultures shape
the ways that indigenous Mexican migrants think about their bodies and "selves,"
about the identities of their colleagues and program participants, as well as the
ways they imagine and implement health programs.

In anthropology, audit culture is defined as "the process by which the
principles and techniques of accountancy and financial management are applied
to the governance of people and organizations—and, more importantly, the

social and cultural consequences of that translation."[4] Within audit culture, quantification and accountability operate as technologies of governance. Together, these technologies influence people, organizations, and even governments to behave in certain ways based on numbers. Among other characteristics, numbers and documentation encourage people to think of themselves as calculating, responsible, self-managing subjects. Shore and Wright explain, "Actors, whether organizations or individuals, are constructed as 'accountable selves' and free agents, who succeed by mobilizing their resources and managing their behavior to optimize 'what counts.'"[5] One manifestation of this culture is what Porter calls "trust in numbers," which creates objective criteria that people, who otherwise would have no basis on which to trust each other, can rely on.[6] For example, foundations know that they can trust the nonprofits they fund if those nonprofits can show them the numbers, including how much is in their bank account at any given time, how much annual funding they receive, how many clients they have served, how many meetings they have held, and, importantly, the results of any audits or evaluations they have received.

Referring to the ways that quantification facilitates a belief in the objectivity of science, Porter's analysis holds not just for social science but for social service. In order to count for services (housing, food, utilities, transportation), people must be counted. They must be countable and accountable. That is, they must turn their identity, activities, and property into a set of numbers in order to both "count" for and "count" on something. One way to do this is to amass the documents that prove their life activities and thus their existence. Even those who are considered undocumented within the United States are charged with collecting and retaining the documents that reflect their existence. If they fail to account for their activities through the appropriate documentation, they miss out on important life opportunities like going to school, renting a house, or getting electricity. Being continually accountable for one's life by continually counting one's activities and experiences is thus vital in a neoliberal society.

One of the consequences of this faith in numbers, however, is both a decrease in personal trust and a move away from localized knowledge. Porter explains that reliance on numbers and quantitative manipulation minimizes the need for intimate knowledge and interpersonal trust while maximizing the need for aggregated information in decision making. "Quantification is well suited for communication that goes beyond the boundaries of locality and community. A highly disciplined discourse helps to produce knowledge independent of the particular people who make it."[7] Rather than capturing the particularities of a person or population, numbers homogenize and universalize experiences. This is what allows bounded categories, such as "indigenous," "migrant," or "program participant," to be meaningful. Homogenizing categories erase the subjective nuances and complexities of what it means to be indigenous or a migrant or a program participant while at the same time converting intimate, local knowledge into aggregates such as the indigenous "population." Such categories obscure the cultural and social differences within and between indigenous peoples and groups while producing and affirming universalizing cultural identities.

Yet, even as the numbers can be reductive and restrictive, they are useful for documenting injustice. As chapter 2 demonstrated, without statistics and other technologies of enumeration, we would have little idea of how many indigenous migrants are in the United States. Nor would we be able to say anything meaningful about the prevalence and severity of their illness burden or their excess death rates. For this reason, numbers are difficult to eschew because they tell an important story about health and vulnerability. Nevertheless, the audit culture with its focus on numbers, accountability, and documentation fosters competition, pitting each player in the numbers game against the other, and the culture of documentation breeds suspicion of those who are either unfamiliar with or not fully invested in it. The paradox for La Agencia is that, as accountability increases and the audit culture infuses their institutional culture, it also creates opportunities for mistrust and uncertainty.

As this chapter argues, institutional cultures, health culture, and indigenous Mexican migrant cultures are coproduced with and informed by all of the neoliberal values of audit culture: accountability, transparency, efficiency, productivity, and documentation. These are measured by particular economic and behavioral indicators, such as the amount of funding received, the number of hours worked, the number of workshops held, and the number of clients served, as well as by embodied indicators like the blood sugar levels and body mass index of their program participants. Good health programming is understood to be accountable health programming, and accountable health programming can be counted and documented by those further up the chain. Nonprofits are accountable to their funders, employees are accountable to their bosses and to each other, and program participants are accountable to the employees. Collapsing the financial and the moral together, the idea of good, accountable health programming thus operates as an ethic shaping both the work of the IHP and the subjectivities of those involved in it.[8] As Luz explained to me,

> Our challenge always, well our obstacle is when we propose how we are
> going to evaluate our programs. A lot of times it's hard to measure them
> quantitatively. Also the methodology that we use has to do more with

the qualitative aspects of the program because what people think is very important to us, if people really think that after having received this training or that program that it helped them or it didn't help them more than if they went to get signed up for medical insurance (Medical) or something else. For me the program would be successful if I go ask the families in individual interviews or in focus groups if their family is better thanks to A, B, or C and not just because we had 50 families use our services in the last two months. For me, that's less relevant but, unfortunately, this brings problems with those who give you the money because they always want to see numbers, numbers, numbers.

Such "governing by numbers" substantially reshapes the ways that indigenous migrants interact with and understand each other, the institutions they work for, the funders who support them, and even their own embodied identities.[9]

Living by the Numbers

My interview with Luz illuminates why indigenous Mexicans do not have bundles of papers documenting their existence. This form of accountability has simply not been part of their daily lives in rural Oaxaca, and therefore they do not prioritize it in California. Because of extreme poverty and the lack of bureaucratic infrastructure in rural Mexico, documentation is difficult to come by. For example, more than 7 million Mexicans lack a birth certificate. The underregistration of births has serious consequences and may even be a cause of out-migration, according to a report from the Migration Policy Institute:

> The under-registration of births in Mexico results in the denial of children's access to education, health care, and legal protection and renders them vulnerable to organized crime, human trafficking, and unscrupulous employers. When unregistered children become adults, they face additional economic hardships and consequences for their civic engagement. There is also anecdotal evidence that disenfranchisement due to nonregistration can lead people who have no formal education and few employment prospects to illegally immigrate to the more opportunity-rich United States, but confront additional challenges there of being stateless.[10]

While the consequences of being stateless in the United States are severe for Mexican migrants, there are political reasons for not wanting personal documentation lying around. As Lynn Stephen writes, migrants "live in a contradictory state of trying to maintain invisibility while simultaneously being the object of significant surveillance at different points in their journey and work experiences in the United States."[11] Given this need to remain invisible even as they are constantly surveilled, migrants leave identifying documents behind in Oaxaca so as to maintain anonymity if they are caught by immigration authorities. The few documents they do bring, such as vaccination and examination records generated by Mexican migrant health programs, such as Vete Sano, Regresa Sano (Go Healthy, Come Back Healthy), are often left behind in backpacks ditched in the desert at the last minute so migrants can blend in once they reach the other side or have been taken by the border patrol and never returned.[12] As Berta told me, "When I tried to cross the border the first time the border patrol caught us and sent us back. The good thing is that we didn't carry our money in our backpacks, we carried it apart, and they [the border patrol] took them [our backpacks] and threw them away. They had chips and meat in them, and they threw everything away." Once they arrive in the United States, migrants working in the agriculture sector are often moving around following the crops. Lugging cumbersome paperwork is neither practical nor possible.

The fact that indigenous migrants do not document their lives does not mean that their lives are not documented in the United States, however. Indeed, one of the main things promotoras do for their health program participants is fill out forms that document all of their relevant life activities. For example, when I asked a Mixtec focus group participant about the differences between the role of the U.S. promotoras and the role of those in Mexico, she said, "Well, I don't know, for me there are not so many papers over there as there are here. Here you have to apply for Medical and for who knows how many programs that you want to have. You have to apply and fill out forms. There are not so many programs that help you [over there]." The availability of the promotoras and their knowledge of the papers required for the various systems was a huge relief for the community. As Alicia's husband, Jeronimo, the Mixtec leader in Greenfield, explained, "Whatever document, whatever written request, or whatever information they need, they go running to La Agencia because they help them fill out the papers. They feel like it's easy there." A female program participant standing by chimed in: "We feel better because if we have a paper and we fill it out with a private company, they will probably charge us. If we have a problem we just have to call them [the promotoras] so they will tell us what we have to do and then they tell us and that's it. It's a big help to us." One of the reasons that people have to fill out so many papers, I was told, is because there are more social programs in the United States than in Mexico. "There's more help here than over there."

The promotoras encourage indigenous migrants to participate in other documentation activities, as well, in order to increase the services available to them. For example, there was a huge campaign by indigenous activists to get Oaxacan migrants to participate in the 2010 Census and to self-identify as both Hispanic and Native American. In 2020, La Agencia's employees created videos in different indigenous languages encouraging people to participate in the census. Because Census Bureau data are used to define the characteristics of populations served by various programs and the characteristics of governments and organizations eligible to receive funds to provide those services, documenting the demographic changes in the migrant community matters: it could result in more services and resources directed toward indigenous Oaxacans.[13] With this in mind, La Agencia employees told people across the state of California to use the Census as a way to document their existence. The result was that indigenous migrants became a recognizable demographic. According to anthropologist Lourdes Gutiérrez Nájera, "Although contemporary large-scale indigenous migration to the United States from Latin America began in the mid-20th century, indigenous migrants were not counted before 2010."[14]

There have also been significant efforts by those affiliated with both the Binational Indigenous Resistance Movement (BIRM) and La Agencia to get birth certificates for migrants who never had documentation on either side of the border. Both organizations have worked closely with the Mexican consulate and with their affiliates in Oaxaca to help people file the necessary paperwork to certify their place and date of birth. I witnessed one meeting they had organized in the Central Valley where parents waited patiently for hours, sitting on plastic folding chairs in a dimly lit room, to speak with a Mexican official about their getting their birth certificates while their kids sat outside on the curb playing Mario Kart on their hand-held Nintendos or running around the parking lot to burn off excess energy.

The need to document everything from birth until death in the United States was illuminated in my conversation with Luz:

Rebecca: Based on what you are saying, it seems that you have to document your entire existence?

Luz: Oh yes! For example, there are a lot of older people that have never had a birth certificate and this is part of what our sister organization [BIRM] is doing in Mexico. They are helping families start the process to get their older family members a birth certificate that they have never had in the United States. There are people that have died without one, and it has never

been an obstacle. For example, [my colleague] Jorge's grandmother arrived
here, and the woman did not even know when she was born, nor did she
have a birth certificate. OK? And they don't believe us when we arrive at a
social service office and what's the first question that they ask you? What is
your birth date? I mean, from the beginning they are looking for you in the
computer and [they say,] "What is your birth date? How are you not going
to know your birth date?" [And I respond,] "Señora, you are talking about
a culture in which papers, numbers, dates are not what is important. You
are, you're important because of other things, not because of when you were
born or your age." So this is a huge challenge that I think is going to play a
role, is already playing a role in whether people get services or not and not
only health services but services in general.

As Luz's comments demonstrate, the audit culture of service provision is bound
up with the accounting culture of immigration, the numbers culture of the
United States, and the broader quantification of everything.[15] So pervasive and
taken for granted is this quantified culture that it becomes almost unbelievable
that there are people in the world who don't operate from its imperatives.

The assumption that everyone is or should be living their lives by the numbers, and the disbelief that occurs when they don't, was illuminated in one of
La Agencia's cultural sensitivity workshops. These workshops, described in
more detail in chapter 5, seek to make service providers more sensitive to indigenous behaviors and norms. During the question-and-answer period at the end
of one of the workshops, a woman stood up and, explaining that she was a nurse,
asked what she could do to get indigenous parents to give their children their
medication. She said that she had tried a number of strategies with one family,
including educating the parents on the importance of giving their child the
medication on a consistent schedule, providing them a container with days of
the week accompanied by a drawing showing which pill should be given at what
time, and even making regular visits to their house to make sure they were com-
plying. Exasperated, she said that her next step was to call Child Protective
Services because these parents were being negligent and putting their child in
harm's way by not medicating him on a regular schedule.

In response, Jorge, one of the presenters and the assistant director of La
Agencia at the time of the workshop, asked if she had assessed whether the parents knew how to tell time. He explained that because indigenous Oaxacans
predominantly live in rural, agricultural communities, they live by sun time,
not clock time. This means that many of them cannot read a watch or a clock,
so no matter how many ways you tell them to give the medication on a consis-

tent basis, it is unlikely that they will succeed. Upon hearing this response there was a murmur across the room as everyone processed the novel insight. The look on the face of the nurse who had asked the question slowly changed from exasperation to surprise as she grappled with her own cultural assumptions about the universal capacity to operate on clock time. Jorge's important intervention put into stark relief for the audience the fact that people often take for granted their own ways of thinking as "normal," leading them to categorize others as abnormal, pathological, and even criminal. The nurse's failure to recognize how subjected she had been to a culture of quantification and to the imperatives of constant and ubiquitous numerical accountability led her to blame indigenous culture for what she had only been able to understand as intentional neglect and abuse.

Where Indigenous Culture and the Audit Culture Meet

Within La Agencia, the audit culture is overlaid with a perceived need to increase the accountability of and to indigenous communities. Because of a history of corruption, theft, and fraud in indigenous organizations in Mexico, indigenous leaders living in the United States have called on indigenous activists to be accountable to the people they serve. Such calls for accountability were made by Rufino Domínguez Santos, a pre-eminent leader in binational indigenous movements and an influential figure in the indigenous migrant community. It was clear that Rufino was preoccupied with the idea that indigenous people must work within the law. He was especially concerned that nonprofits not be viewed as acting politically or lobbying for particular issues, as that would be against the law, as he understood it. While it is true that nonprofits cannot campaign on behalf of political candidates, they can engage in some lobbying, but because the stakes were so high for indigenous migrants, Rufino did not want indigenous organizations to be seen as unaccountable.

Writing about the internal crises and future challenges for indigenous organizations, Rufino describes the need for written accountability in indigenous communities:

> Leaders of a financially successful organization may, however, be tempted to misappropriate the organization's resources, especially if these leaders lack the wherewithal to support their families. There are many honest leaders, but we must also recognize that there is also corruption and the abuse of authority, and we must speak out as a first step toward finding a solution to the problem. Accountability, decision making by consensus, teamwork and delegation of responsibilities are the sacred

principles that guide authorities in indigenous communities, and these
are the practices that must prevail in indigenous organizations. Part of
being accountable to the bases is informing the community in writing
about the leaders' and staffers' activities and the overall plan of work.[16]

Rufino's admonition to his indigenous brothers and sisters in California was
taken to heart by La Agencia's staff, some of whom felt that the need for accountability and an unwavering trust in numbers superseded trust in their word.
Each week the promotoras on the Central Coast had to write a weekly report
and submit it to the main office. Otherwise, as they told me, "they won't believe us that we did all of this work." The weekly reports would include the
number of people helped by each promotora, the number of workshops each
held, the number of participants in each workshop, and the number of hours
that each employee had worked. This weekly exercise of accountability was repeated by all of La Agencia's employees across the state. The weekly reports
were then compiled by Luz and used when writing reports to funders. They
were also used when writing grants soliciting future funds. The weekly activity
reports thus offered proof of La Agencia's past successes and showed that they
deserved further investment.

The need for written accountability to the main office influenced the work
of the two Central Coast promotoras, who were afraid that the main office would
think they were not working hard enough. Given that they worked in programs
funded at the whim of foundations, they also feared they would lose their jobs
if they couldn't produce the numbers. This led them to constantly compare their
numbers, each trying to outdo the other in the amount of work they did, the
hours they were on the job, and the resources members of their ethnic community received. Their anxiety shaped interactions with their program participants,
who they regularly entreated to attend their workshops. Framing their pleas in
terms of "mutual support," the promotoras would tell people from their respec-
tive ethnic communities that if they didn't show up, the main office would think
that the promotoras weren't doing their jobs, and then the participants might
lose access to them. This would mean that the promotoras couldn't help the
community to solve their problems or fill out their papers anymore. If people
wanted to keep the promotoras, then they needed to "support" them by showing up whenever they organized community activities. So great was the worry
that at one point I even witnessed Jeronimo encouraging people to attend his
wife's workshops so that staff in the main office "would not think that the promotoras are just sitting around not doing anything."

Because they never knew if they would have jobs past the next grant cycle or if they were meeting the main office's standards, Berta and Alicia perpetually tried to increase the number of people they helped each day and the number of people that attended their workshops by enticing them with food and other resources. They even jealously guarded their participant lists so that the local clinic, who asked for the contact information of IHP attendees, couldn't poach people from their programs. Citing the lack of reciprocity from staff at the clinic ("They won't tell us who they talk to, so why should we tell them who we talk to?"), Alicia interpreted the staff's secrecy in terms of competition for funding rather than a HIPAA (Health Insurance Portability and Accountability Act) violation, which it undoubtedly would have been had the clinic revealed their patients' information. Underlying all of the promotoras' efforts was the presumption that the more successful of the two would be less likely to be let go in the event of budget cuts.

Their ongoing sense of precarity led to tensions in the toll booth. For example, on the days when the Salvation Army held its monthly $20 voucher giveaway, each of the promotoras competed for the only telephone in the office. They wanted to call people from "their" community to let them know about the vouchers since it was first come, first served. Between frantic calls to people on her program participant list, Alicia explained to me that "last month all of the Triquis got the vouchers since they are always in the street." Her implication, which is based on long-standing ethnic tensions between Mixtecs and Triquis in Oaxaca, was that because Triqui women are looser—what Alicia called *callejeras* (streetwalkers)—they learn about the voucher giveaway sooner and get there faster. It was true that, because Triqui women were often without transportation when their husbands were in the fields or had migrated to other communities to work, they would walk everywhere. They were walking the streets because of a lack of resources not a lack of values. Nevertheless, Alicia wanted to be sure that this time the Mixtecs, who in her opinion were good women staying in their houses where they belong and minding their own business, did not miss out. She also wanted to be sure that the Mixtec community knew that she was responsible for getting them additional resources and that, when it came time to attend community activities that she organized, they would owe her. Indeed, she would remind them of this during the health workshops, saying that they needed to keep attending the educational activities she offered because she had been helping them to get needed resources. Occasionally, Alicia stayed on the phone for so long during the voucher giveaways that Berta would have to walk down the street and, with her own money, use the pay phone to call her *raza*, a term she frequently used to refer to the Triqui community.

Tensions over resources and numerical accountability in the office spilled over into many of the IHP activities on the Central Coast. For example, the promotoras knew they needed to bring food and drinks to the community meetings or else, as they explained, "people will not show up." Yet, they also knew there were limited funds in their program budget to pay for these snacks. This led to a dilemma before every health workshop: Who would pay for the snacks, would they be reimbursed, and, if so, how? Taking ownership over the Mixtec community as she would her own family, Alicia insisted that each person provide the snacks for her own ethnic group. That way, if the money was not reimbursed, she could justify it in terms of mutual support. She took great pride in choosing the snacks that, to her mind, most closely corresponded to the tastes and nutritional needs of the Mixtec population. Such thoughtful decision making would please her people, she reasoned, and would make them want to keep coming.

Berta, by contrast, insisted that the two women, and sometimes even myself, should *cooperar* (pool our money) to pay for the snacks, no matter which group was attending. She reasoned that we should all take responsibility for all of the program participants, no matter their ethnicity. This line of argumentation was undoubtedly informed by the fact that she had much less cash on hand to pay for the snacks and thus could not afford to wait for reimbursement from the main office or to purchase the snacks without reimbursement. If we all pitched in, her financial burden would be lessened and her *raza* would not suspect that she was unable to take care of them. Her food choices were, as a result, most often driven by financial rather than nutritional concerns.

While disagreements about who should pay, who should be reimbursed, and what kind of snacks to buy occurred regularly, the real tension occurred whenever there was leftover food and water from a workshop. These would be stored in the tiny toll-booth office and vigilantly surveilled by each of the promotoras to be sure that the other woman was not doling out water or fruit to "her" people if she had not paid for them. Cases of leftover water bottles would be symbolically stacked next to the desk of the promotora who purchased them. When a client from one ethnic group asked if she could have a water or a snack purchased for members of the other ethnicity, the two promotoras exchanged tense looks. Because resources were scarce for the promotoras, for the program participants, and for the IHP, they paid close attention to how much they spent, how much their *gente* (members of their community) consumed, and how much people from the other ethnicity took from their stash. Resentments between the two manifested in each one of them gossiping to me about why the resources were justifiably meant for the exclusive use of "her" people.

Overall resource scarcity in indigenous communities and the precarity that is driven by grant funding became personalized over time and carried over into other aspects of their job. On one occasion the promotoras had to travel three hours to the Central Valley office for a meeting about immigration laws. La Agencia staff had asked a lawyer to discuss legal issues affecting migrants in the United States and to give an overview of proposed legislative reforms, including a much-hoped-for amnesty. Alicia offered to give Berta a ride, but Berta's husband, Francisco, didn't want her to go without him. Francisco was notoriously possessive and did not like his wife going to strange places unaccompanied because, as he once explained in response to Luz's teasing about his watchful eye, "If something happens to her what am I going to tell her family? I am responsible for her." Because Alicia did not like Francisco, who she thought was too controlling, she said that he could not go in the same car with her. This caused a huge scandal in the main office. Francisco didn't have a license and had to ask a friend to drive them, causing them to be very late to the meeting. In addition, the two promotoras ended up driving separately, which led to two costly travel reimbursements rather than one as anticipated. The financial tensions in the toll booth thus led to financial frustration in the main office, both of which caused interpersonal tensions between staff members. While these tensions could be easily attributed to historical ethnic tensions, which were undoubtedly part of the dynamic, they were largely informed by the demands of the audit culture and its requirements of accountability, documentation, and individual responsibility. Indigenous culture and audit culture became entangled, and, in a context where every penny literally counted because of resource scarcity, job insecurity, and financial uncertainty, everyone was worried about the bottom line.

Paying to Work

The kinds of resource insecurities that were evident on the Central Coast were also evident during La Agencia's strategic retreat. The retreat, which happened every three years, brought employees, board members, and allies from across the state together in a beautiful mountain setting. In the rolling hills above the Central Valley, staff members met in wooden buildings to revisit the mission and vision of the organization, outline the strategic program areas, and discuss the future of La Agencia. One of the retreat sessions was focused on the financial situation of the organization. As had been expected for some time, the executive director and one of the board members described the dreaded reality that the budget was not sufficient to keep all of the employees. A conversation about the need to increase the budget while decreasing expenditures ensued. One of the ideas that was floated by a promotora from the Central Valley office was for employees to put a percentage of their paychecks back into the operating budget in order to keep the organization afloat. Everyone would make less money, they reasoned, but they would still have a job, and La Agencia would still be able to help the community. After some discussion it was agreed that everyone would give back 5 percent of their income in order to keep the organization running.

I was a board member and adviser to both La Agencia and BIRM at the time, and this discussion upset me. I could not understand how such a precarious and poorly remunerated workforce could stand to lose a portion of their income like that. More devastatingly, this proposal was tantamount, in my mind, to paying to work rather than getting paid to work. It followed from worrying trends in the market wherein employees, notably in the University of California system where I was completing my PhD, were being furloughed and having to purchase their own computers and paper. The signs of paying to work seemed to be everywhere as more and more budgets in academia, in industry, and in the nonprofit sector were being shifted from "hard" money to "soft" money, and employees were guaranteed work only on short-term, flexible contracts. This shift was putting valuable community organizations, like La Agencia, and their employees in positions of extreme vulnerability and financial uncertainty, and it would certainly have effects on the communities they served.

Pushing back against the proposal, and holding back tears of fear and frustration driven by my own sense of moral and financial responsibility to La Agencia, I suggested that giving part of their pay to the organization that had been established to support them and other indigenous migrants like them was not a viable solution. It was like a snake eating its own tail insofar as the organization could not continue to exist on such a financial model, and its employees could not afford to give up a portion of their already meager pay. Nevertheless, my concerns were overridden by the leaders of both BIRM and La Agencia, who likened the proposal to *tequio*, a form of unpaid labor in indigenous communities that is organized for collective benefit. Such collective or communal work has a long history in Oaxaca where it is used, as Jorge once explained, "to keep our communities running." Although *tequio* was exploited under the colonial authorities as a way for indigenous peoples to pay tribute to the crown with their labor, it is now seen as a core, defining feature of indigenous community sovereignty and indigenous Oaxacan culture.

Reinterpreting free labor, or what from my perspective was the equivalent of paying to work, as *tequio* illuminated the ways in which indigenous culture and the audit culture became almost indistinguishable in the work of La Agencia. Indeed, as is well known, and as we were reminded at the retreat, organizations that have a track record of showing responsibility by effectively managing their money, including by keeping at least two months (often more) of their operating budget in the bank, are those that are most likely to be funded by scrupulous foundations. Having cash on hand, rather than in their employees' pockets, would enable La Agencia to secure further funding, which presumably would then allow their employees to go back to full pay. If everyone put their *gota de agua* (drop of water) in the bucket, then everyone would benefit. Much like the mutual support that the promotoras asked from their communities, the reinvestment solution would keep La Agencia running by making the people who benefit from it responsible for its success. I never could decide whether *tequio* or the neoliberal imperatives of the audit culture were at work in that approach. What was clear to me from this discussion was that accountability to funders, "owning" the problem, and indigenous sovereignty looked surprisingly similar.

Making Accountable Subjects

In addition to the staff's regular reports to the main office and the reports from the main office to the funders, another method for accountability was soliciting feedback from program participants about the kinds of health information they had seen or would like to see in La Agencia's workshops. In order get anonymized feedback, La Agencia occasionally hired a program evaluator to conduct focus groups. The results would be compiled in a report that could be furnished to potential funders as justification for new or continued support. Participant feedback also came from collaborations with local civic leaders and service providers. The promotoras would invite their program participants to community meetings held by their collaborators so the participants' voices could be heard and they could, at the same time, learn new information.

One such meeting took place when Maria Santiago, a city council member at the time and a vocal advocate of the indigenous community in Monterey County, wanted to conduct a focus group with Mixtec women in order to find out about their health needs. Maria was known to the indigenous community through her efforts at monthly town-hall meetings sponsored jointly by the local police department and the small city where the promotoras worked. These informative meetings, meant to address community concerns and educate the

indigenous migrant community about laws and services, were generally organized and attended by Maria along with another city council member, Jesus
Sanchez, and led by the local chief of police. The town-hall meetings were
meant to show that the local government was accountable to its citizens, but
also to teach those same citizens that they were accountable to local laws and
norms.

Maria was a trusted health resource for the La Agencia promotoras because,
in addition to her civic work, she worked at a local rehabilitation center for drug
and alcohol addiction. Thus, when she asked the promotoras if they would
invite some female participants from the IHP to be part of a focus group so she
could hear their needs and convey them back to the city and to her nonprofit,
they were happy to comply. Many of the public workshops were attended by
both indigenous men and women, but the men often dominated the conversation. The promotoras saw Maria's focus group as an opportunity to hear the
unfiltered voices of the indigenous women they served.

Seven Mixtec women attended the focus group, which was held in the city
council chambers. Maria and her assistant had prepared ten focus group questions in advance and handed them out to each woman as she walked in. They
had also written them up on large white sheets of paper in the front of the room.
The questions had to do with health care problems, access, and resources, as
well as what the city could do to address these issues. My experience of the
Mixtecas was that, in comparison to the Triqui women, they generally spoke
up in group situations and shared their opinions and views. On this day, however, they were very quiet and spent a lot of time looking around the room or at
their feet. The first question, "What are the biggest health problems you and your
family face in the community?" was initially met with silence. Eventually one
woman spoke up and explained, "The problem we have is that we don't know
if we are sick because we don't go to the clinic, and we don't go to the clinic
because we only think about working and because they charge high prices in
the clinic." No one else responded to the question.

Maria asked the second question, "When someone in your family has a
health problem, how do you try to solve it? Where and whom would you go
to?" Again, only one woman answered, explaining, "Although we get sick, we
don't want to go to the doctor, and instead we buy pills at the store because at
the doctor they ask us for insurance and we're embarrassed. Because they ask
us for it we don't go. We just use the syrup that they recommend to us within
our own community. When we don't know where to go or what to do we go to
our [local indigenous community] leaders." The third question, "In the last year
or so, what changes have you seen in regard to heath issues in your commu-

nity?" went unanswered, as did a series of subsequent questions asking for comparisons between the present and the past: "Is it easier or more difficult to solve your health problems now than a year ago? Why? Do you feel you have more knowledge in obtaining information about necessary resources now than a year or two ago? What kind of progress do you see in obtaining health resources in your community? What has made it better in accessing health resources, and how can it continue?" All of the questions asking for feedback on the role of the City in providing health resources also went unanswered: "Do you feel more confident interacting with the City and other resource agencies? What has improved the relations with the City and the resources you have received, and how can this be improved even more?"

One question did get responses: "What problems remain in regard to health care?" To this, one woman answered, "Health insurance. When I go to the doctor, they don't even want to know why I am there. They just want to know if I have health insurance." Another woman interjected, "You feel bad because you come from work and you don't even have money to pay the doctor." In response to these comments, Maria began asking if the participants were familiar with the local and state health insurance programs, in response to which she was told, "We don't know about other places, we only know about this place [La Agencia]." When asked if there was anything else they wanted to share, one person mentioned that it would be good to have a place to go to get free screenings. Another woman explained that she is always working when the local free food distribution at the food bank occurs, so she is unable to access it. Maria confirmed that from now on she would have the food bank put aside a bag for her and would personally hold it so the woman could come and get it. With that, the focus group ended.

Maria's focus group sought to solicit opinions and feedback from residents on the services provided by their local government in order to make those services more responsive and accountable. From the perspective of La Agencia, these interactions are important because they bring together two of the organization's concerns: health and civic engagement. As discussed in chapter 2, getting indigenous women actively involved in issues of concern to them has been one of the goals of both La Agencia and its sister organization since the beginning. But this focus group was important for reasons beyond that.

First, it reveals that health insurance, above all else, is the primary concern of the focus group participants. Going to the doctor is difficult because of work commitments, but even when the women do go to the doctor, it is expensive because they don't have any insurance, and they don't have health insurance because they don't have documentation that proves their citizenship. The problems that brought them to the doctor in the first place are ignored until the question of whether they have insurance coverage has been resolved. Because undocumented migrants in the United States are prohibited from obtaining health insurance except in emergency circumstances, their options for care are limited. This information goes against what I heard from some nonindigenous community health workers, who said that indigenous people don't have a culture of going to the doctor but instead depend on their own cultural traditions, such as taking herbs and making teas. In fact, women in this focus group had experience with clinical care and wanted the same access in the United States as they had in Mexico. As one woman, exasperated that such a powerful country as the United States had such an inaccessible health care system, explained to me, "In terms of the clinic, the hospital, here everything is very expensive and this is a powerful country, the number one country in the world. Mexico is a poor country but you know IMSS (the Mexican Social Security Institute) is free. In a lot of little towns there is no clinic, but where there is a clinic it's free."

Not only is clinical care prohibitively expensive in the United States, but many migrants also fear receiving clinical care or presenting themselves at a hospital for treatment given the stories they have heard about the consequences of authorities catching them without documents. These consequences include arrest and deportation, disqualification for future benefits, and the up-and-coming practice of "medical repatriation" in which hospitals pay the expense of deporting undocumented and uninsured patients in order to avoid incurring more costs associated with their care.[17] This means that even though they may want to go to the doctor, many migrants either wait until their health condition is emergent or they forgo care altogether.[18]

Contrary to what I had been told by clinic workers, then, it was not because they had different cultural beliefs that indigenous peoples did not use health care in the United States. It was because the culture of documentation in the United States prevented them from having insurance or from having employment that would offer them insurance. As one woman explained to me during an interview, "Over there [in Mexico] in the clinic or in the Social Security [IMSS] if you're black or white or whatever you are it's free, not because you don't have papers or because you're a gringo or because you're Japanese [you can't go]." And another added, "Because in Mexico it's different because if we know that we're very sick we know how much they are going to charge us. Yesterday I arrived here from Mexico and I punctured my foot. I went to the clinic and they asked me if I had health insurance. I had to pay the visit and then they gave me another appointment in a month. What if I die in a month?" Lack of clinical access in the United States puts indigenous migrants in a hopeless situation: they go to the doctor because they feel bad, but then they feel bad for going to the doctor because they can't pay or they don't have the documents to get treated. In the end, they just stop going to the doctor.

The underlying complaint of the women in Maria's focus group revealed that their lives are regulated by considerations that have little to do with indigenous culture: they cannot get to the doctor because of work, they are unable to see the doctor because of lack of money, and their identities and bodies are not valued unless they have been recognized through a documented health insurance plan. This regulation exposes them to increased risk because they cannot access the services that will ensure their health and well-being. As a consequence of this, and acutely aware of their vulnerable situation, the women are concerned with acquiring health insurance as a means for accessing health care. This concern was highly evident that day. Although the representative sample is quite small, this finding adds to the growing evidence that health insurance is a primary concern for Mexican migrants generally and for indigenous migrants specifically.[19] It also shows that the imperatives of audit culture to document and represent people's identities as a series of numerical representations prevent indigenous migrants from exercising their "duty to be well" even as they try to be responsible health subjects.

This focus group is also important because it provides a space for a population generally silenced in public spaces by gender and racial discrimination. Yet, when given the opportunity to speak, the Mixtec women hardly participated. Their silence could have been a consequence of their unfamiliarity with Maria, or even of the formality of the city council chambers. I heard many times from the promotoras and from La Agencia staff that indigenous migrants were intimidated by "experts" and feared doing or saying the wrong thing around them until they had established trust, or *confianza*. Indeed, I had been pushed to the front of the group on many occasions to speak on behalf of my indigenous colleagues because, as they told me, "you're a *gabacha* [white person] and they will believe you."

On the other hand, when they did feel strongly, as in the case of health insurance, some of the women began speaking up. Because of this, I suggest that the silence of the participants has as much to do with their self-understandings as with the context or interlocutor. By this I mean that the indigenous women do not understand themselves as at-risk health subjects. They are not in the habit of scrutinizing all aspects of their lives for danger or of calculating their individual actions and decisions based on possible health risks in the past or the present. Comparing past health behaviors with present health problems was not something that came easily to them. If anything, Maria's focus group was teaching them to think in this way, challenging them to exercise an active citizenship around their health needs. Indeed, I had experienced a similar response when I tried to conduct my own focus group with the Mixtec community. I asked the participants what themes were important to them: Nutrition? Navigating the health system? Making better health decisions? One woman responded by saying, "Well, you have to tell us. You have more words and more experience."

If given the opportunity, indigenous women will participate in collective decision making in their home communities, but the decisions most often have to do with local politics and not the quantification and comparison of personal health issues over time or the collection and comparison of community health data.[20] The imperative in the United States to constantly reflect on one's state of health is not as predominant or pervasive in rural Oaxaca. Not only is this imperative unfamiliar, but the idea that one should constantly be checking on one's state of health is scary for some. More than once I heard that women didn't want to go to the doctor because they didn't want to know if something was wrong with them. While the women in Maria's focus group, like those in mine, were unprepared to answer questions about changes in their individual health or about dynamics in the community's health over the last year, they were clear that the idea of going to the doctor was terrifying because if they find out that they are sick with something serious and don't have health insurance to address it, they are stuck. As the woman in the diabetes prevention group discussed in chapter 1 told me, *mejor no voy* ("It's better if I don't go").

Maria was not the only one to struggle unsuccessfully to glean information from the indigenous community using the focus group method. I observed a health program supervisor from the Monterey County Health Department attempt to engage Mixtec men and women by asking what the health department could do to provide more health information and services to the indigenous community on the Central Coast. Her questions went unanswered. An evaluator for La Agencia from Bolivia also attempted a focus group to ascertain indigenous community needs regarding health issues. She found it extremely difficult to engage the group participants and lamented later that the focus group method was not very useful in her evaluation.

The Oaxacan tradition of public gatherings in which community issues are discussed and decided collectively led me to believe that the focus group method would be successful. Indeed, there is a long history in Oaxaca of *usos y costumbres* (customary law), in which the community selects leaders, decides on community duties, and generally runs itself. As I observed over time, however, health focus groups were not necessarily a useful method for getting unfiltered feedback. This is not because indigenous Oaxacans don't have an opinion or a voice but because these focus groups assume a particular self-understanding that comes from living in a risk society. In a risk society, "the self becomes a 'reflexive project' that involves the abandonment of a concept of the life course being shaped by tradition and certainty in favour of one that is a series of passages involving at each stage the calculation of risks and opportunities."[21] The questions raised and the concerns illuminated in health focus groups are based on a health subject who understands that her health is perpetually "at risk" and can articulate what she is "at risk" for (obesity, high blood sugar, the flu, allergies, asthma, and so forth). The women in the focus groups must first learn that they are at risk and then learn their individual risks before they can articulate them. As the woman in the diabetes prevention workshop discussed in chapter 1 told me, she learned about diabetes from the promotoras. The information they gave her "has stayed in her head." Now she worries about what is in her blood and how high her sugar is, but she, like many in my focus groups, said they never worried about such things before.

The understandings of risk among indigenous Mexicans, who are linguistically isolated from many media outlets and have not been exposed to as much preventive health education, are quite different. This does not mean that, as Luz once told me, "they don't have a culture of prevention." Instead, the values and ideas that shape that culture are not based on an incessant cost–benefit calculation. Examples abound in the indigenous community of preventive action. For example, indigenous people engage in prevention by observing the *cuarantena* (the forty days after giving birth) to prevent postpartum complications, tying a red band or a bracelet with *ojo de venado* (a velvet bean referred to as deer's eye) around a child's wrist, covering a child with a shawl, keeping a child dirty or putting spit on the forehead in order to prevent *mal de ojo* (the evil eye), avoiding extreme temperature changes or exposure to *aires* (cold air), and not getting up too fast after eating to avoid *empacho* (indigestion or constipation), to mention only a few.[22] This sense of prevention does not always translate into a context or language dominated by allopathic medicine, nor does it involve a constant self-monitoring of weight gain or loss, caloric intake, A1C levels, blood pressure, or other numerical indicators of health, however.

The comments of the Mixtec women who did speak in Maria's focus group show that their actions have been guided neither by calculations of health risks or opportunities nor by the quantification of their health, at least not in Maria's terms. Certainly, the choice to migrate involves great calculation of risks and opportunities. When it came to discussing their health, however, these women did not express their needs in these terms. For example, as their comments indicate, they do not go to the doctor when they are sick, nor do they know of health insurance programs that would make doctor's visits accessible to them. Instead, they go to fellow community members. This response does not demonstrate the loss of traditional commitments and support relationships that scholars have argued occurs in a risk society.[23] Although one woman in the group was concerned to find out what she might be at risk for, none of the women indicated having been engaged in the "processes of endless self-examination, self-care, and self-improvement" called for by neoliberal health imperatives. Indeed, no one could articulate whether health issues in the community had improved over time, or even if their own individual health problems or health knowledge had improved. In a society that has shaped the quantified health movement and in which health has become the business of everyday life, this lack of preoccupation with quantified health indicators is remarkable.

Despite the participants' inability to articulate what they might be "at risk" for, to use Maria's terms, or whether the risks they are exposed to had changed over time, the focus group did serve a pedagogical purpose insofar as it taught the participants how they *should* think about themselves, their health, and their lives. At the same time the indigenous women were giving information, they were also learning what information to give. Thus, while soliciting information from indigenous women about their needs in order to develop accountable programs and policies, Maria was at the same time teaching them what it is possible to know and want given the context and their condition as undocumented, migrant workers.

The focus groups were therefore teaching indigenous migrants to assume a more entrepreneurial and empowered health subjectivity, one in which their voices counted and in which they began to think about their bodies and their health in calculative terms, under the guise of accountable governance. While accountable governance assumes a population that already has an idea or that feels they should "own" the problem of their health, in my observations the focus group participants were gathering ideas on what problems they should and could "own" in the United States based on the expectations and questions of the researchers and evaluators they encountered.

The fact that indigenous communities in California were learning to "own" their health problems, while simultaneously being accountable for their behaviors and activities, was clearly illustrated in an external evaluation of La Agencia's programs. A particularly pervasive audit practice, external evaluations are an important mechanism of accountability for nonprofits because they show efficacy at multiple levels. For example, they demonstrate the effectiveness of community programming to the foundations that fund them; they show the organizational leadership of the nonprofit how well their frontline employees are doing their jobs; and they show the frontline workers how well the community is responding to their efforts. The success of La Agencia's programs was documented in an external evaluation that was conducted from 2004 to 2007. The evaluation reported that, of twenty-eight program participants interviewed, 75 percent of those who had attended La Agencia's health workshops expressed that the topics provided had affected their personal and extended family's lives either directly or indirectly. In terms of their direct impact, most of the interviewees indicated that they changed some of their daily practices, including how they washed their clothes, how they cooked, and what they drank. The workshops had not only changed those who attended them, but as the evaluation states, participants also reported that the effects of La Agencia's programs extended to family members who had not attended, but who received some of the preventive health information from their siblings or parents who had. As a result of hearing what was being taught by the promotoras, family members and friends changed their lifestyles, and some even went to the clinic to be checked for diabetes and asthma. As the evaluation demonstrated, accountability for indigenous health both trickled out to the community and, through the evaluation process, trickled up through the organization to its funders.

Conclusion: Culture Counts

Drawing from the idea of the audit culture, this chapter has shown how instrumental practices of enumeration, documentation, and accountability are operating within the IHP. Beyond ensuring transparency and efficiency, these techniques also function as technologies of governance and power shaping organizational and individual behavior and indigenous self-understandings. As Shore and Wright have argued, actors within an audit culture, whether organizations or individuals, are constructed as "accountable selves" and free agents, who succeed by mobilizing their resources and managing their behavior to optimize "what counts."[24] When indigenous migrants do not or cannot fulfill the demands of the audit culture by optimizing their health, their voices, their time, their resources, and all of the other things that both "count" and can be counted, then they are blamed, disbelieved, and, in extreme cases, disciplined and punished. When they do succeed, however, they are rewarded with vital resources.

The goal of this chapter has been to show, on the one hand, that there are more cultures, values, norms, beliefs, and behaviors at work in the IHP than just the culture of Oaxacan indigenous migrants. The values of the audit culture, including accountability, productivity, and efficiency, have all contributed to the ways that La Agencia employees have made decisions, interacted with each other, and even negotiated their wages. These values have also shaped the ways that nonindigenous service providers view indigenous migrants and understand themselves. As with the nurse who never imagined that the "problem" with the indigenous family had to do with her own assumptions about what it means to live by clock time, many service providers cannot imagine or envision a world outside their own experiences. This leads them to disbelieve that there are other ways of being and acting in the world and to become suspicious of those who don't act like them. Unfortunately, this inability to imagine the world otherwise leaves indigenous migrants in a difficult position. They are expected to "own the problem" of their health, but that problem often has more to do with the cultural expectations and accounting demands of others than with their own behaviors and self-understandings.

On the other hand, this chapter has sought to show the ways in which indigenous cultures and the audit culture are sometimes mutually reinforcing, entangled almost to the point of being indistinguishable. This view aligns with the assertion of Shore and Wright that audit culture is not monolithic or uniform. Rather, as they explain, "audit practices work in diverse ways and have diverse meanings and ramifications in different contexts."[25] Audit practices and practices of indigenous sovereignty begin to resemble each other within the daily operations of La Agencia. To return to an idea introduced in chapter 1, scientific ideas and beliefs about health and medicine are coproduced with the representations, identities, discourses, and institutions with which they interact. To the extent that the audit culture infuses health epistemes and practices within the IHP, it also shapes indigenous subjectivity. Indigenous cultures and the audit cultures of health philanthropy are therefore evolving together. This dynamic is captured by anthropologists of the audit culture: "Setting performance indicators and assessing against benchmarks and best practice are instruments designed to make organizations more 'accountable' to funders, government, stakeholders, consumers, and the public. While they render individuals and organizations more 'legible' to external experts, there is a coercive dimension to that accountability: organizations must represent themselves in terms of the narrow, predetermined script of expert assessors, in what Strathern calls the "tyranny of transparency."[26] In the case of La Agencia, however, rather than extracting the opinions of the participants in order to develop accountable programs and policies and to write successful grants, the focus groups were instead teaching participants what to think and worry about with regard to their health. These groups, meant to extract information, were actually providing the information they wanted to hear, thereby indoctrinating indigenous migrants into the audit culture. This iterative pedagogical process ultimately acts as a technique of governance and power under the guise of accountability, transparency, and empowerment.

Because La Agencia employees have witnessed so many interactions in which they or their program participants have been disbelieved, blamed, or punished for acting outside dominant norms, they have developed a cultural sensitivity workshop in which they invite audience members to understand and embrace their idea of what it means to be indigenous. As part of the organization's bidirectional strategy for bridging the differences between indigenous and nonindigenous populations in California, the cultural sensitivity workshop aspires to make service providers more empathetic and sensitive when dealing with indigenous migrants by opening up their worldviews to other ways of being and acting. Chapter 5 discusses this workshop and draws out its implications for intervening on the cultural and political imaginaries of nonindigenous service providers and for La Agencia's efforts to create a healthier and more welcoming environment for indigenous migrants.

Cultural Sensitivity Training and the Cultural Politics of Teaching Tolerance

> As a form of passive resistance, this invented tradition is both salvation and damnation. For just as it strengthens the Indian community, so also does it become a stigma of the oppressed.

A Clash of Cultures

On January 11, 2009, in Greenfield, California, Marcelino de Jesus Martinez, a thirty-six-year-old indigenous man from the Mexican state of Oaxaca, was arrested and later charged with procuring a child for lewd and lascivious purposes, aiding and abetting statutory rape, and misdemeanor child endangerment. The child implicated in the matter was Mr. Martinez's fourteen-year-old daughter, whose marriage to eighteen-year-old Margarito de Jesus Galindo was said to have been arranged in exchange for $16,000 and hundreds of cases of beer, soda, wine, Gatorade, and meat.[1] The arrest was made when Mr. Martinez went to the police to report that his daughter was missing. As the police investigated, they found that the girl had not run away, but rather had voluntarily gone to live with her would-be husband, apparently with the consent of her father.[2] Her father had purportedly sought the help of the Greenfield police to get her back because the agreed-upon sum remained unpaid. The father's concern was quickly overshadowed, however, by what came to be labeled a "clash of cultures" by the local police chief, Joe Grebmeier.

The "clash" Grebmeier was referring to involved the cultural norms of the Triquis, the indigenous group that Mr. Martinez belongs to, in which girls in their early teens commonly marry adult men. The practice of "underage marriage" is less common in California, where the legal age for marriage is eighteen except by parental consent.[3] In addition, the arranged exchange of food and drink, as well as a large sum of money, led to allegations that the father had sold his daughter, a provocative spin that caused some discussion of whether this case constituted human trafficking. It was later determined that it was not trafficking because there was consent on the part of the girl to be married.[4] In addition, the goods and money to be exchanged were meant to constitute a dowry and supplies for the wedding celebration, not a fee for the sale of the daughter, as many newspapers were reporting. Chief Grebmeier explained that, despite the legal and social implications in the United States, "It never occurred to anyone involved that they were breaking the law."[5]

This situation drew the eye of federal agents because there was the possibility that some federal laws had been broken.[6] Federal immigration agents determined that Mr. Martinez was in the country without authorization and, as a consequence, would be subject to deportation proceedings after the local prosecution.[7] Emotions were further heightened by the report that while she was away from her parents, Mr. Martinez's daughter had engaged in sexual relations with Mr. Galindo. The case went global as media sources reported the story to audiences as far away as Australia and Croatia.[8] In response to the media reports, online commenters seethed with anti-immigrant sentiment. One comment read, "Which dead Americans ss# [social security number] is he using to stay in this country? Automatic deportation."[9] Another commenter wrote, "Where is the mother in all this or did they sell her too???? What a moron!"[10] Amid the sensational reporting and emotionally charged comments, one person illuminated the greater challenges presented by the situation, writing, "Such a sad story in some ways, and yet what can one do laws are written to fit local customs. So what happens when cross migration of cultures happens. This is all part of a bigger melting pot than any of us had ever imagined."[11]

Affirming Social Hierarchies through Cultural Narratives

The Greenfield case is significant not only because it provides insight into the challenges that Oaxacan migrants confront when they come to the United States, but also because it demonstrates how a cultural explanation about indigenous migrants is the readily available framework for making sense of the issues in the case, even though there were significant U.S. legal, political, and economic

factors at work. As the public response evidenced, allegations against Mr. Martinez brought to the surface anxieties nascent in the long-standing debates on immigration in the United States, anxieties that hinge on seemingly stark differences
between "us" and "them." These debates alternately feature immigrants (especially if they are undocumented and brown) as terrorists threatening the public's
safety, as welfare magnets or job stealers threatening the public's economic well-
being, or as criminals, carriers of contagious diseases, and purveyors of unhealthy lifestyles constituting a threat to the public's health and welfare.[12] These
readily available cultural narratives have become so pervasive that it is difficult
to find a media narrative that doesn't engage at least one of them. Such narratives
have also infused the imaginary of conservative academics. For example, political scientist Samuel P. Huntington, former professor at Harvard, has suggested
that the particular cultural threat posed by Mexican migrants, a threat he calls
the "Hispanic challenge," penetrates beyond any one sector and, according to his
view, threatens the very cultural identity of the nation.[13]

The Greenfield case drew on these cultural anxieties and also reinforced
the idea that indigenous people live a "traditional" existence that has not caught
up with the twenty-first century. The elements highlighted in the case by both
law enforcement and the media (child endangerment, sex trafficking, unauthorized immigration) played on historical fears of the cultural "other" as backward, uncivilized, and impoverished. The case painted a picture of indigenous
Mexican men as so lacking in modern sensibility that they were willing to sell
their underage daughters for money and groceries, as sexual deviants whose
pathological personalities threaten not only their own offspring but also the
moral fabric of the community and, by extension, the nation. This was not the
first time that such an image was used to depict the Triqui in Greenfield.[14] Further, the indigenous women involved in the case were depicted as lacking
agency, voice, and identity, as mere pawns to be shuffled between uncaring, lascivious indigenous men and the protective custody of the U.S. state. The facility and rapidity with which Mr. Martinez was demonized, and the extent of
media coverage his case received, point to the tension between rhetoric and reality in a society that prides itself on being both multicultural and color-blind.

The media attention that the Greenfield case garnered shows how pervasive and politically convenient the trope of "backward cultural others" is
for making sense of complex social issues. Indeed, this cultural trope serves as
the dominant interpretive framework for indigenous migration. However, it
obscures the normative role that social organization plays in defining who and
what is culturally backward or, by contrast, culturally civilized (or simply "cul-
tured"). The focus on indigenous cultural practices masks the ways that social

hierarchies are produced and reinforced through cultural narratives. For example, Jordan and Weedon have argued that social divisions, marked by differences in appearance, behavior, and speech, are largely secured through culture—that is, through belief systems, social rituals, ideologies, and other modes of intersubjective thinking and acting.[15] In addition, "the relative domination of various groups is partly secured and reproduced through the practices and products of cultural institutions," including language, family, media, education, the law, and religion. As the Greenfield case highlights, indigenous forms of social organization are seen as an affront to nonindigenous cultural institutions and also, to echo Huntington, as a threat. The Greenfield case provided an opportunity for nonindigenous observers to reaffirm their own social status and standards by demonizing Triqui culture.

The negative media attention that Triquis received as a result of Mr. Martinez's actions did not go uncontested, however. Indigenous scholars and activists pushed back, issuing a public statement condemning the sensationalism and the negative portrayal of indigenous culture. At the same time, nonindigenous anthropologists who had worked closely with the Triqui asked provocative questions about the cultural practices of nonindigenous people. For example, Seth Holmes asked, "Who are Americans to say that their marriage practices are better than the Triquis, especially when fifty percent of U.S. marriages end in divorce?"[16] These contestations played an important role in denaturalizing hegemonic forms of social organization and the cultural narratives they rely on. As Jordan and Weedon explain, "Battles to transform the nature of the educational system, to shift the pattern of control in the national media, to rewrite history and to reconstruct human beings" are all efforts to displace or deconstruct dominant cultural constructions, meanings, and values.[17] Similar to the demonizing cultural narratives that affirm social hierarchies, resistance to domination is also rooted in cultural narratives and personal experience.

Cultural Politics and/as Embodied Politics

La Agencia's employees are acutely aware of the insidiousness of cultural tropes about indigenous migrants. Over the years, they have witnessed overt and covert racialized dynamics in which indigenous migrants were treated poorly because of cultural assumptions by those working in health, social service, and law enforcement. For example, in Greenfield, California, a Triqui man was pulled over and had his car impounded for "looking" illegal. When the police officer stopped him he said, "I can tell you are illegal. . . . I can tell you have no papers."[18] In yet another case of misunderstanding in Greenfield, a police officer was called to an event in which, according to an INS media spokesperson, "a tragedy may have narrowly been avoided." The case involved a recently arrived Triqui man who disrobed at a local laundromat to wash the only set of clothing he owned.[19]

They have also observed the consequences of miscommunication and misinterpretation of indigenous behaviors, which have occasionally resulted in the incarceration and deportation of some of their indigenous friends and clients and, in extreme cases, even death.[20] For example, in Los Angeles, California, Manual Jamines, a K'iche'-speaking Guatemalan man, was shot twice in the head by Los Angeles police officers because he did not respond to their commands in Spanish.[21] In Oregon, Santiago Ventura Morales, a Mixtec man, was accused of murder because he would not look police officers in the eyes, among other purported signs of guilt. Morales, who was not fluent in Spanish, remained incarcerated for four years before his case was reopened and his conviction overturned.[22] Morales's lawyer, Paul De Moriz, illuminated the issues at stake in the case when he wrote, "Linguistic and cultural differences can unfairly penalize immigrants thrust into the cauldron of the American justice system."[23] One of the jurors, who supported the guilty verdict, went on to say he wished Ventura had been sentenced to death, qualifying his desire by saying, "We don't need so many of 'em running around here."[24]

Uninformed cultural assumptions are also pervasive in health institutions. For example, in Oregon, Adolfo Ruiz Álvarez, a Triqui man, was confined to a mental institution and kept sedated for two years before being released. Officials thought that Álvarez was mentally ill because he was of Mexican origin but did not speak a language that was intelligible to anyone he was interacting with.[25] Once it was discovered that he spoke Triqui, he was released. In another instance, one of La Agencia's Mixtec *promotoras* (community health workers) working in the Central Valley was accused of human trafficking by clinical staff when she accompanied a pregnant woman to her medical appointment to interpret for her. As the promotora explained to me, they called the police "because they thought I was trafficking babies."

In another highly publicized case in Mississippi, Cirila Baltazar Cruz, a Chatina woman from Oaxaca, was charged with child neglect and endangerment because she did not have baby diapers, formula, or a crib and because she struggled to speak Spanish and did not speak English.[26] The Mississippi State Department of Human Services ruled that Baltazar Cruz was an unfit mother in part because her lack of English "placed her unborn child in danger and will place the baby in danger in the future." One of the Binational Indigenous Resistance Movement's (BIRM's) associates interpreted in the case and explained to the court that indigenous women use cloth diapers, breastfeed, and cosleep. The interpreter also made the case that Chatino is as valid a language as Spanish, even if it is spoken by fewer people. Given her intervention, the case was eventually overturned, the baby was returned to her mother after two years apart, and, with the help of the Southern Poverty Law Center, Baltazar Cruz successfully sued the hospital and state employees that had persecuted her.[27]

Hoping to minimize, if not altogether end these traumatic situations, La Agencia developed a cultural sensitivity training, titled "Understanding the Oaxacan Indigenous Culture," that provides important information about the culture that shapes the lives of indigenous Oaxacans in Mexico and in the United States. The term "cultural sensitivity," as they employ it, connotes a level beyond competency or awareness; it calls for providers to consider and respond appropriately—sensitively—to the cultural differences of indigenous peoples. For La Agencia staff members, critical reflection on these differences distinguishes "competency" from "sensitivity." La Agencia's cultural sensitivity trainings are meant to complement the direct services and health information they provide to indigenous Mexican migrants through the Indigenous Health Project. Their hope is that by educating service providers, many of whom are health care workers, about indigenous culture while also educating service recipients, all of whom are indigenous, about health, the interactions that result will be more respectful and effective.

Using the framework of cultural politics, this chapter examines La Agencia's cultural sensitivity training. "Cultural politics," according to Nina Glick Schiller, "refers to the processes through which relations of power are asserted, accepted, contested, or subverted by means of ideas, values, symbols, and daily practices." Because La Agencia's training frames and thus in some sense determines the meanings of what it means to be indigenous, their efforts to transform the ways that service providers think about indigenous migrants are an important mechanism for contesting relations of power and dominant narratives. The trainings present the "public face" of indigenous Oaxacans to audiences who often have very little knowledge of the differences between indigenous and mestizo Mexicans and who have little understanding of where indigenous people come from or how they live in Mexico. At the same time that these trainings provide a new way of thinking about indigenous migrants, they also provide an opportunity for service providers to accept or contest this new knowledge. The analysis in this chapter is informed by the following questions: What are the cultural politics at work in the cultural sensitivity trainings? How do they work to mitigate racism and promote indigenous health? Do they achieve their goals?

Providing insight into the cultural politics of cultural sensitivity training is important, not only for La Agencia but for all those who seek to teach
cultural competency, humility, and tolerance. As Jordan and Weedon assert,
those who study cultural politics are concerned with the ways in which culture
is used to legitimatize the social relations of inequality so they can work to transform these inequities.[28] The transformational potential of cultural competency is
what draws many practitioners to it as an approach for working with diverse
populations. As I found, however, developing competency about a cultural
"other" is the easy part. Cultural self-recognition, on the other hand, is much
harder than it seems because nonindigenous people tend to think that they have
no culture, that their way of being simply reflects what it means to be human.
This perspective creates a fundamental challenge to the antiracism work that La
Agencia is trying to promote as part of the IHP and forces indigenous activists to
frame their approaches in less politicized and more palatable ways.

Representing the Oaxacan Indigenous Culture: La Agencia's Cultural Sensitivity Training

It is a typically cool, sunny morning in a small town on the Monterey Bay where
we will be giving a workshop on cultural sensitivity. As the crowd of social
workers, nurses, law enforcement officials, city administrators, and other interested stakeholders gather in the community conference room, my indigenous
colleagues and I huddle together around the podium to plan the schedule and
timing of our presentations. We decide that La Agencia staff members Jorge and
Luz will introduce themselves and describe the services that La Agencia offers
in different cities throughout California. Then the two promotoras working in a
nearby town will introduce themselves. I will go next and discuss the history
of indigenous colonization and contemporary indigenous migration to the
United States, focusing on the social determinants of indigenous health. Then
Jorge and Luz will discuss what it means to be culturally and linguistically sensitive when providing services to or interacting with indigenous Mexican
migrants in the United States.

By the time the introductions start there are at least seventy-five people
seated. More slowly trickle in, quietly closing the door behind them as they scan
the room for an empty seat. Jorge, a Mixtec man from San Miguel Cuevas, a small
village in Oaxaca, begins. He explains that La Agencia was formed in 1993 as
an outgrowth of an indigenous social movement and in response to the needs
of indigenous Mexican migrants, many of whom were not fluent in Spanish and
did not understand the services and systems in the United States, and all of

whom regularly had their labor rights violated while working in the agricultural fields of California. He describes how La Agencia established itself as a non-profit offering interpretation services, teaching leadership skills, and informing farmworkers about their rights.

Now, with over two decades of experience, Jorge explains, La Agencia has expanded its services to include health, nutrition, literacy, and a variety of other activities, including teaching indigenous dance and language. After giving a broad overview of their services, Jorge introduces the two promotoras involved with the Indigenous Health Project on the Central Coast. The first, Berta, boldly steps forward to welcome everyone. A round-faced Triqui woman with long black hair and dark eyes, she is wearing the traditional clothing of Triqui women from western Oaxaca, a *huipil*—a loosely fitting red and white dress with color-ful threads running horizontally within the fabric and a brightly colored ribbon sewn vertically down each side and capping the sleeves. Although her dress reflects the tradition of her home community, Berta does not usually wear a *huipil* in California. She has worn it on this day because she had been asked to demonstrate the cultural traditions of the Triqui. The oldest of five siblings, Berta had left Oaxaca in her sophomore year of high school to come to California with her father. She learned to speak Triqui working in the agricultural fields of Cali-fornia and had learned about indigenous Oaxacan traditions by accessing radio and TV shows in the United States that were not available to her in Oaxaca. As she admitted to me, "I've learned more about myself, my home state, and life in Oaxaca living in the U.S." As Berta stepped aside, Alicia timidly came forward. She, too, was wearing traditional clothing, which for Mixtec women is a white, cotton blouse or loose-fitting dress with brightly colored embroidered flowers. A short woman with shoulder-length hair, Alicia often embraced the latest fash-ion, which meant that for the workshop she was wearing jeans and wedge heels with her floral blouse. Alicia smiled, revealing several silver-capped teeth, and greeted everyone in Mixtec.

Like Berta, Alicia was the oldest of five siblings. She had attended school until the sixth grade and was married by age fifteen. Her husband was the locally elected Mixtec authority. As his wife, she gleaned a lot of respect from her *gente* (fellow community members). Unlike Berta, however, Alicia had spoken Mix-tec since she was a child. The difficulty of attending school in Spanish was one of the main reasons she gave for dropping out at such an early age. She and her husband had significant resources in California, including a van to give farmworkers paid rides to the fields. Because she had more social and economic capital than many in her community, she was not that invested in being a community health worker "where you have to work all the time and be away from your family." She often talked about returning to the fields so that she could work beside her husband and be home with her kids in the evenings.

After the two promotoras had been introduced, Jorge introduced me as a member of La Agencia's board of directors and a researcher studying indigenous migration and health. As I cued up my PowerPoint, I explained to the audience that I had been studying health programs for indigenous Mexican migrants in California. In that process, I found that understanding indigenous health in the United States requires having a better historical understanding of where indigenous Mexicans are coming from and why they come to the United States. This history, I explained, offers important insights into the structural vulnerabilities that indigenous people have experienced for over five hundred years, first at the hands of the Spanish colonizers, then at the hands of mestizo Mexicans within Mexico, and then from the American empire as it has exercised increasing economic and political control of rural communities in Mexico through trade policies like the North American Free Trade Agreement. These historical events, I explained, are social determinants of indigenous health. Understanding them provides insights into the health of indigenous people before and after arriving in the United States. After finishing my presentation, I ceded the podium to Jorge and Luz to deliver the same cultural sensitivity workshop I had seen them deliver on multiple occasions throughout California.

Understanding the Oaxacan Indigenous Culture

La Agencia's cultural sensitivity training touches on the following: a definition of cultural competency, the demographic profile of indigenous people in Oaxaca, indigenous history, traditional medicine, family values, migration patterns, living conditions in California, and organizing efforts. It is meant to provide a broad overview of indigenous Oaxacans, including where they come from, who they are, how they act and why, and how they live and solve their problems in the United States. There are usually two presenters, Jorge Garcia, a Mixtec from San Miguel Cuevas, and Luz Villanueva, a mestiza woman from the state of Mexico. Each had lived in the United States for more than eight years at the time of the presentation in Watsonville, and each spoke excellent English.[29]

The overall goal of the training, as the presenters explain, is to "strengthen collaboration between La Agencia and health and social service providers in an effort to improve the well-being of indigenous communities and educate providers on the functioning of the U.S. health and social systems." This goal is described to participants at the conclusion of the training, and the presenters then offer tips for health and social service providers, suggesting that they should "train all staff to be more sensitive in providing service to indigenous people, especially if they do not speak English or Spanish; provide interpreters in indigenous languages whenever needed; and take into account the cultural background of the indigenous migrants when judging their behavior." The entire presentation is meant to provide an interpretive framework for understanding indigenous culture and behavior.

The definition of "culture" used in the presentation is taken from Spector: the "sum of beliefs, practices, habits, likes, dislikes, norms, customs, rituals, and so forth that we learn from our families and years of socialization."[30] Drawing from this definition, the presenters open by describing indigenous customs and rituals. Jorge discusses the political organization of the community, called *usos y costumbres*, also known as customary or normative law, in which the practice of *tequio* (unpaid labor to benefit the entire community) is central. This form of civic governance dates from the pre-Hispanic era and continues today, Jorge explains. The custom of *tequio* is for males over eighteen to assume *cargos* (duties) in the community for a fixed period of time (from one to three years). The point of *tequio* is "to make community projects happen." It is defined in the presentation as "collective work for the benefit of the whole village." This indigenous custom is obligatory, not voluntary, and so men who are living in the United States need to return to their community of origin to fulfill their *tequio* or risk being ostracized from their hometown.[31] Jorge discussed the added burden the men's absence puts on their families in the United States as husbands, sons, and fathers return to Mexico to pay their service to the community with their labor.

One of the rituals discussed in the workshop is the Day of the Dead, or *Día de los Muertos*. This holiday is described as a day to "remember and show appreciation for loved ones who have passed away." In particular, the presentation cites the Zapotecs as maintaining this tradition by decorating altars with food, alcohol, and marigolds to welcome their dead back. Jorge, who had previously returned to Oaxaca at least once to welcome his grandmother who had passed away, explains, "On November 2, we think that the spirits of our loved ones come back and taste the food." This tradition involves leaving the door to the house open so the spirits can easily re-enter the home. Many indigenous migrants, like Jorge, feel the need to return to their communities of origin in order to open the door for their loved ones, and they lament that, with increased border security and rising airfares, this is becoming an impossibility. Jorge was very close to his grandmother, and it pained him that he lacked the financial resources and time off from work to return to visit her every year.

Another ritual introduced in the presentation is the Guelaguetza, a cultural and social celebration that, according to the presenters, has been practiced since the pre-Columbian era. The word "Guelaguetza" comes from Zapotec and means gift or offering. The celebration shows gratitude to the Creator for the good harvest and allows participants to give or share food, music, and dance.[32] The presenters explain that indigenous migrants are now teaching indigenous dance to other migrants in order to preserve the tradition of the Guelaguetza, and there are currently numerous Guelaguetza celebrations throughout California.

The primary custom emphasized in the presentation is the use of traditional or indigenous medicine. The presenters take turns explaining that, among indigenous Oaxacans, it is believed that external agents (supernatural, human, and nonhuman) cause illness. They describe how sickness can result from strong emotions (such as fear, anger, and jealousy) or evil spirits. Babies are especially vulnerable to strong emotions, and mothers often do not let strangers hold or come near their newborns. Examples of ethnospecific illnesses, such as *coraje* (anger), *nervios* (anxiety or stress), *susto* (fright or soul loss), *empacho* (indigestion), and *mal de ojo* (the evil eye), are provided but not defined. Jorge and Luz also explain that indigenous healers have specialties, just like allopathic doctors, and in addition to their role as healers, they are seen as community leaders and protectors who possess divinatory and prophetic skills. Their healing rituals include the use of medicinal plants, prayers, ceremonies, and card reading. The purpose of the healing rituals, according to them, is to restore the equilibrium of the sick person, who may be too hot or too cold or, in the case of *susto*, may have lost their spirit.

The presenters explain that people may go to an allopathic doctor and also seek help from an indigenous healer. Because clinical services are less accessible, however, and rural medical units in Oaxaca are often short on medications, traditional healing or "folk" medicine is the first line of defense. Drawing on the work of medical anthropologist Bonnie Bade, who has called this practice "transmedicalization," Luz explains that indigenous migrants do not abandon their cultural beliefs in the United States but instead mix them with the health services available here, often seeking help first from a traditional healer and then from an allopathic doctor or clinical practitioner.[33]

As Luz described this mix-and-match approach, I recalled a conversation I had with Alicia in which we discussed her decision-making processes for pursuing a healer. Intimating that Berta, the Triqui promotora, was carrying around too much anger and jealousy and that it was influencing her baby's health, Alicia explained the remedy:

If the baby's diarrhea is green, we go to the *curandero* [folk or traditional healer]. If she has a fever and is hot on the palms of her hands and the bottom of her feet, and she is vomiting, then we go to the *curandero* because that is a sign that someone said she is beautiful baby and gave her *mal de ojo*. If I take her to the clinic like that, they will do a blood and urine test and tell me nothing is wrong, that my daughter is normal. But, I know that my daughter is sick and she needs to be cleaned with an egg. That alone will cure her. If it is a yellow or brown diarrhea, we go to the clinic and they can help.

Because she attributed her baby's illness to her coworker's strong feelings, Alicia decided that once she had the baby cleaned by the *curandero* she would not bring her to work with her anymore. Instead, she would take her lunch breaks at home where she could see her baby and breastfeed her.

After discussing several of the rituals and customs practiced by indigenous Oaxacans, the presentation introduces family and social values. Jorge and Luz emphasize the importance of nuclear and extended family, especially when it comes to providing mutual support, caring for children, and helping other family members to meet their needs. They highlight the importance of elders as prominent community members and the value of women as those who take primary care of the family. Because parents work so much in the United States, the presenters explain, they have a difficult time preserving this cohesion.

The discussion of values also highlights the indigenous perspective regarding child-rearing and the importance of teaching children responsibility. This information is interlaced with information about cultural and, ultimately, legal clashes in which well-meaning parents take their children to work in the fields or leave underage children to care for their younger siblings and are subsequently punished for breaking child labor laws or for neglect. Child discipline is the primary example the presenters give to demonstrate how cultural differences can lead to legal repercussions. They explain that discipline in indigenous families can include not only yelling but also physical punishment, which is considered child abuse under U.S. law but which is not perceived as such by indigenous parents.

They also describe how parents feel a sense of helplessness in the United States because their children often threaten to call 911 if the parents attempt to discipline them. The lack of disciplinary authority leads children to do what they want, which often results in them spending a lot of time in the street and possibly joining a gang. This information was echoed in a conversation I had with Alicia's husband. He told me that indigenous children know how to call 911, and they do so whenever their parents ask them to do something they don't want to do. "When the police come, they believe the children. That's why parents are losing control of their families. They are afraid the police will deport them or take their children away." Jorge and Luz also discuss the indigenous custom of girls getting married at a very young age. They explain that this can create legal difficulties for indigenous migrants and can result in moral clashes between legal authorities and indigenous parents, as happened in Greenfield. Legal frameworks in the United States consider this to be statutory rape unless the couple is married, and a minor can only marry with the consent of her parents. If the parent's consent to the relationship but there is no legal marriage, the parents can still be held legally accountable.

The final point the presenters make about culture has to do with language and communication styles. They explain that "indigenous people do not express their ideas straight to the point. They need to contextualize their problems and experiences." For example, if they started experiencing headaches after they fell down by the river, they need to give the details of where, when, and how they fell since these important contextual clues might help with diagnosis and treatment. Further, they need to feel confidence and a sense of trust in the person with whom they are communicating. Luz explains that when communication is not effective, it can result in further family complications. For instance, when indigenous children refuse to learn their parents' language of origin and grow up speaking English or Spanish instead, this can lead to intrafamily divisions. In extreme cases, poor translation or no translation has resulted in the institutionalization of indigenous migrants. In one case cited in the presentation, a couple spent a night in a Fresno jail because the hospital staff were convinced they were trying to kill their child when they did not follow medical recommendations but instead, because of a lack of understanding, did exactly the opposite.

To say that one speaks Mixtec or Triqui is not enough information for adequate interpretation, the presenters explain. One must also know the region and village from which the client originates in order to know whether the interpreter speaks the same dialect. The presenters stress the need to make materials visually and verbally accessible to a population whose reading level often does not exceed the sixth grade, to have service hours that correspond with community needs, and to use community leaders or gatekeepers to build trust and rapport with clients in order to effectively communicate with them.[34] Given the centrality of communication, the presentation concludes by stressing the importance of finding an interpreter who speaks the same language and dialect of the person receiving services and reminding the audience that offering interpretation services is required by law for any service provider that receives federal funding.

The Politics of Indigenous Culture

Leave aside for the moment the fact that the cultural sensitivity trainings essentialize Oaxacan indigenous identity and render indigenous culture, which is used in the singular, as a homogeneous and fixed set of beliefs and practices, despite at least seventeen different languages being spoken in Oaxaca, each with its own dialects, and the fact that at least one of the indigenous staff members had learned to become "more" indigenous upon arriving in California. It is important to analyze the discourse and politics the presenters are promoting through their choice of topics. While explicitly discussing culture, these trainings also elaborate on conceptions of indigenous rationality and the relationship of indigenous people with nature, life and death, and self and community. In sum, through their discussion of culture, the presenters describe how social and political power is conceptualized in indigenous communities.

At the same time that the training presents a sketch of indigenous culture as if it were a fixed reflection of indigenous "truth," the presenters also will it into existence through their desire to have service providers understand their indigenous clients in this way. That is, in the process of discussing the culture and therefore the politics of indigenous Oaxacans, they simultaneously create this culture and politics as real. In so doing, they themselves are offering a political representation of the world into which they hope to entice the service providers. Or, at the very least, they are inviting the providers to understand that there are "other" ways of living, and that the providers should be sensitive to these other ways. Such a wishful enactment is part of their struggle to have providers understand indigenous Mexicans outside cultural stereotypes or superficial media narratives. Foregrounding this epistemic and hermeneutic "pluriversality" in their trainings is an example of what Mignolo refers to as "decolonial thinking," or imaging a world in which many worlds can coexist.[35]

What "truth" or reality are they presenting? What are its implications? Embedded in the discussions of *tequio* and of the primacy of family we see a community politics that puts the group before the self or individual. The "logic" informing this is "if the community well-being is secured, then my individual well-being will also be secured," thereby reinforcing the idea and practice of collective solidarity and interdependence through "a qualitative economy of communal reciprocity."[36] This sense of self contrasts with the Western, liberal notion of self and subjectivity, which privileges the individual over the collective. Families' willingness to be separated from their fathers, sons, brothers, and husbands, who must return to their hometowns for the good of the community and in order to stay physically connected to the social body through their labor, demonstrates the strength of this community spirit. The presentation reveals Oaxacan ethics and politics in a comparative frame. Luz explained that indigenous Oaxacans "have a moral obligation to participate. The primary identity in indigenous communities is communal and collective. The U.S. is very individualistic in comparison."

Immigration scholars have begun to discuss the fact that many migrants now pay someone else to fulfill their *tequio*, or they have a family member, even a female, complete their *cargo* because the emotional, physical, and economic cost of the travel home is too high.[37] This commitment reflects the importance of supporting the community even when one is far away. Despite this changing trend, there are some men who return to their communities of origin. Indeed, I met a Mixtec man while he was serving his *tequio* on the Comité de Salud (health committee) in San Miguel Cuevas, Oaxaca.[38] His job was to open and close the clinic every day. He fulfilled this *cargo* while his family was living just down the street from my mom in Fresno, California.

The discussions of indigenous medicine and the Guelaguetza provided in the workshop show the importance of living with and as part of the earth, rather than dominating it. The celebration of the fruits of the earth, especially corn, demonstrates the value of nature in the ongoing survival of indigenous Oaxacans, and the embodied dances that celebrate nature point toward the symbiotic relationship between humans and the earth. The use of plants to heal disease is also a testament to indigenous people's relationship with nature in which each has a role to play in the survival of the other. Thus, this cultural discussion forwards a role for humans in which they do not control or dominate nature, even their own, a perspective antithetical to that of the modern, liberal subject who believes that nature, including their own, is and should be controlled by humans. In order to secure their health and well-being, and as part of their cultural constitution, indigenous Oaxacans look outside themselves to the social and material world for the support necessary to keep on living. Indeed, this ties into the prior theme, in which the well-being of the collective body comes before that of the individual body.

As Luz and Jorge explain, this belief is also reflected in indigenous etiologies, which see external rather than internal agents as the cause of illness. For this reason, indigenous healers, employing eggs and other natural elements as diagnostic tools, must use their divinatory powers to assess the possible social or historical factors that have caused the person to become sick. Their questions to the patient, which are generally very few, are focused on the social history of the person prior to their falling ill. Consequently, the indigenous diagnostic process often entails a long discussion in which the patient recounts everything that happened to her before she got sick. This is in contrast to clinical doctors, whose many questions, reflected on health history forms filled out prior to a visit, often focus on the biological history of the patient even when the categories are labeled "social history." This clinical approach is concerned with patient confidentiality and encourages both the privacy and autonomy of patient decision making, by contrast with the indigenous healing process that reflects a "cultural safety" model of health by incorporating the family and members of the community, who can be present for both the diagnosis and the healing ritual, and can participate in decision making for the patient.[39]

According to the presentation, malevolent spirits are not the only spiritual influences in indigenous social life. Relatives who have passed away continue to have a presence in the lives of their family members. This is most evident on the Day of the Dead. The ongoing presence of spirits, malevolent and benevolent, challenges the idea that only living human beings are actors in the world. Indigenous understandings of community and family are capacious enough to extend not only across national borders but across lifeworlds. This provides a particular political vision of citizenship and belonging in indigenous communities, a belonging not exclusively identified with geography, the state, the materiality of the body, or a teleological conception of time.

In sum, the perspective of indigenous culture forwarded in the cultural sensitivity presentation emphasizes—and thereby proposes—a particular political and ethical relationship between self and other in the effort to foster life and well-being for indigenous people. This relationship puts the social body before the individual body, assumes a relationship of equality and symbiosis with nature, and incorporates a variety of actors—living and dead, human and nonhuman—in its conceptions of life and health. Such collective solidarity reflects a social contract that ensures, to the extent possible—notwithstanding globalization, government repression, and intracommunity violence over land disputes—both the physical and economic security of community members in communion and relation with other living beings. It is a politics based on ecological solidarity and communal reciprocity. The goal of the presentation is to reinforce the importance and value of "alternative" or "other" visions of life that inhere in indigenous culture so that, in their interactions with Oaxacan migrants, service providers can be more sensitive and, as Jorge once said in a pertinent mistranslation from Spanish, "sensible."[40] Luz summed up the goal of the training when she said to the service providers, "If you think, 'I am right, I have the truth,' the only thing you'll accomplish is putting a barricade between you and the client. If you come from a positive perspective, they will be open. You would feel the same."

Power and Tolerance

The cultural sensitivity presentation goes a long way toward providing those in the helping professions with the necessary tools to improve services for their Oaxacan clients. As a result of attending the training they will know that Mexicans are a multilingual and multiethnic population. They will have some understanding of indigenous social and political organization, and they will be able to recognize, if not fully understand, some Oaxacan healing traditions. The fact that the presentation is delivered by a Mixtec migrant from Oaxaca and a Mexican migrant woman, sometimes with the presence and participation of other indigenous staff members from La Agencia, reinforces its cultural and linguistic relevance and offers embodied proof of the cultural differences that are discussed.

Despite its powerful testament to the strength, beauty, and resilience of Oaxacan cultures, however, I suggest that the presentation also works in tension with La Agencia's goal of promoting cultural sensitivity because it essentializes indigenous Oaxacan culture and also reinforces a distinction between self and other in which the service providers remain the point of reference against which the indigenous "others" are necessarily defined. In other words, it helps service providers become "competent" about a group of people, presented in static and essentializing ways, while never asking audience members to grapple with the ways that their own lives and behaviors are structurally tied to the lives and behaviors of the migrants they seek to help. Audience members are asked to be tolerant of the cultural differences and to become competent in what those differences are, but they are never challenged to understand how those differences are historically, politically, economically, and even culturally produced. Significantly, the presentation obscures the fact that the audience members also have traditions, norms, and practices—that is, cultures—which they neither have to reflect upon nor explain to indigenous migrants. The explanatory process only goes one way, and it only focuses on the ways that indigenous people are culturally different from nonindigenous people. It does not point out how nonindigenous people, too, have historically informed cultural particularities, among them the pervasive belief that indigenous peoples are a culturally static population whose members mostly live a backward and uncivilized existence until or unless they assimilate to American culture.

Wendy Brown's discussion of tolerance is useful here. Brown argues that when tolerance is mobilized as a political discourse concerned with designated modalities of diversity, identity, justice, and civic cohabitation, all of the things that La Agencia's cultural sensitivity training is concerned with, it marks those subjects to be tolerated as inferior, deviant, or marginal vis-à-vis those practicing tolerance.[41] She explains, "Almost all objects of tolerance are marked as deviant by virtue of being tolerated, and the action of tolerance inevitably affords some access to superiority."[42] Not only does the discursive appeal to tolerance produce as inferior those subjects to be tolerated, it also depoliticizes this production by naturalizing cultural difference and then arguing that social inequality, subordination, and conflict are based on ahistorical and essentialized cultural differences. In other words, the "culturalization" of difference operates in the same way as the racialization of difference. Brown explains, "Tolerance discourse reduces conflict to an inherent friction among identities and makes religious, ethnic, and cultural difference itself an inherent site of conflict, one that calls for and is attenuated by the practice of tolerance."[43]

Applying this to the cultural sensitivity training, we see that La Agencia's presentation depoliticizes the historical and political sources of what is presented as an essentialized indigenous cultural difference, thereby politicizing the "difference" itself rather than its modes of production. This depoliticization leads, in turn, to calls for tolerance, thereby cementing what appear to be static and bounded cultural differences between indigenous and nonindigenous groups. One example of this ahistorical essentialization is the claim made during the cultural sensitivity trainings that many indigenous migrants fail to make eye contact with nonindigenous people. This is often referred to by La Agencia staff as an indigenous "norm" that should be understood and respected as part of indigenous culture. A historical reading of this lack of eye contact reveals that it is an effect of colonization and should not be essentialized as an ontological feature of indigenous peoples. Rather, it should be understood as a learned survival strategy in conditions of extreme oppression. On more than one occasion this behavior has been misinterpreted by judges and police officers who took it to be a sign that the indigenous person was shifty, untruthful, uncaring, or disinterested. There is, therefore, a lot at stake in deconstructing this so-called norm within the training.

In presenting indigenous culture as static and singular, La Agencia puts indigenous Mexicans in the position of the cultural "other" to be tolerated and situates the service providers attending the cultural sensitivity training as benevolent and altruistic people who are tolerant. Framing the dynamic in terms of altruism has further implications. Insofar as the appeal to tolerance is meant to change the behavior and feelings of the service providers, it makes historically induced suffering a problem of personal feeling, thereby replacing the field of political battle and political transformation—which are the goals of cultural politics—with an agenda of behavioral, attitudinal, and emotional practices. This displacement has consequences, as Brown explains: "While such practices often have their value, substituting a tolerant attitude or ethos for political redress of inequality or violent exclusions not only reifies politically produced differences but reduces political action and justice to sensitivity training, or what Richard Rorty has called an 'improvement in manners.'"[44] At the same time, the diversity that exists within and between indigenous groups is glossed over, and a culturalized (read racialized) indigenous identity is produced, thereby reinscribing a binary between those who are perceived to be ruled by "their" culture and those who rule themselves but enjoy the culture of "others."

This dynamic, in which an essentialized or even obsolete view of culture is used to promote cultural competency, has led to the charge that "cultural competency discourses that define cultures without consideration of power and that do so in stereotypical ways resemble new racism."[45] Following the work of David Theo Goldberg and others who have written about racialized discourse, Gordon Pon explains, "New racism is racial discrimination that involves a shift away from racial exclusionary practices based on biology to practices based on culture." Here, "culture talk" stands in for "race talk." Pon explains that because it uses culture rather than race as the basis for differentiating groups of people, "it is extremely difficult to recognize cultural competency as racism because it discriminates and otherizes without using racialist language."[46] Pon's analysis is in keeping with the critical literature on cultural competency approaches, which finds that they overgeneralize, reinforce stereotypes, treat culture as static, are devoid of both historical context and power analysis, and ultimately offer a Disneyfied version of culture. Not only do these assumptions diminish the complexity of groups of people by homogenizing them as "other" but they also contribute to racially discriminatory views against those groups because they fail to consider and illuminate power relations.

While La Agencia's goal is to mitigate rather than reinforce racism, their way of teaching cultural sensitivity buttresses a binary in which those who rule their nature are perceived as being without or beyond culture, while those who do not dominate their nature but live with and in nature are perceived as being dominated by their culture. This binary bolsters racist thinking among those who already believe that their ideas, beliefs, and daily practices—their cultures—are superior. To the extent that the service providers are the referent in the trainings, they are challenged neither to rethink their own subjectivities nor to provincialize their own cultural particularities. Instead, they are encouraged to reflect on (thereby reinforcing) the cultural "difference" of indigenous Oaxacans

by coming to know how "they" think and act. The subjectivities of service workers as "helpers," "providers," and holders of the "truth" are thereby solidified
and legitimated by the presentation, rather than undone.

La Agencia's explanations of indigenous customs, values, and society
address U.S.-based service providers both as interlocutors and as the population they must convince about the legitimacy and value of indigenous ways of
knowing and being. This dynamic reflects the ways that racialized people have
always had to explain themselves to members of the dominant group, in contrast to those from the dominant group, who do not have to account for their
own behaviors and beliefs. Luz's closing comment, which called for the service
providers to put themselves in the situation of indigenous migrants ("you would
feel the same"), can be seen as a call for social service and clinical workers to
accept this legitimacy. Indeed, it is for this reason that culture is presented in
the workshops as static and "authentic." As Jorge reminded me, if it were to be
more politicized, the audience would not be as receptive.

This reminder came on the heels of my presentation on colonization
and racism that day. I emphasized that racism is not only a significant social
determinant of health for indigenous peoples on both sides of the border but
also pervades humanitarian organizations working to serve them in the United
States. In other words, it infuses the cultural imaginaries of even the most well
intentioned providers. As an example, I described my own experience working
in a nonprofit dedicated to serving farmworker families in and around Watsonville. I explained that I was regularly surprised to hear derogatory comments
from my coworkers, who were predominantly second-generation Latinx, about
our Mexican migrant program participants, many of whom were indigenous but
all of whom were poor farmworkers recently arrived from Mexico. For example, on one occasion we had invited the families that used our services to attend
a clothing drive. Several women showed up with their own children and with
extended family members who brought their children. These women left with
garbage bags overflowing with clothes. As they walked away, my coworker said
to no one in particular, "Did you see how many clothes they took? So greedy!
They're probably gonna sell them."

Over time, and after working in four different nonprofits in Watsonville,
I had come to see that my experience in that organization was not isolated. In
all of the organizations where I had worked, I witnessed coworkers treating the
services, vouchers, and goods we offered as if they were their own, as if the
money to pay for all that we offered was coming directly out of their own pockets. This, of course, couldn't be further from the truth; all of our services were
grant funded, and all of us were poorly paid. In fact, many of us would have

benefited from the clothing drives and the food vouchers ourselves. In my presentation I explained that at the same time that they treated the resources as their own, my former colleagues blamed recently arrived migrants for using those resources. The accusation of greed was made as if migrant farmworkers were somehow, either by nature or culture, greedy. This accusation obscures the ways that inequitable structures make so many of us, including newly arrived migrants, needy not greedy, and the ways that our own employment was dependent on the neediness of others.

Precarious Politics

After our presentation that day, Jorge and I reflected on how everything went. I worried aloud that my part had been too far off topic. In response he said, "You said all of the things I couldn't dare to say in my presentation." His comment reveals the unequal relationship that exists between indigenous migrants and U.S.-based service providers, a relationship that remains unspoken and unaddressed in the cultural sensitivity presentation because it would challenge the cultural hegemony of the audience members and ultimately jeopardize their funding and support. More to the point, it reveals how a cultural politics based on stereotypical ideas, beliefs, and symbolic representations prevents La Agencia from overtly confronting dominant cultural formations. Challenging their audience members in any way is perceived by La Agencia staff as something to be avoided insofar as they need the continued support of those who attend their trainings. They have worked too hard to gain the trust of nonindigenous service providers only to lose it by reminding people that they are structurally and ethically implicated in the injustices that shape immigrant lives and deaths. For example, they cannot remind people that ready access to healthy fruits and vegetables or to cheap childcare and clean hotel rooms, among other things, are possible because of social inequity, nor can they explain that the cultural tropes they are working so hard to undermine facilitate the jobs of social service providers. Fostering hostility toward La Agencia or the indigenous migrants that they help would not be a desirable outcome. Indeed, one of the purposes of the trainings is to make the audience members more empathetic, supportive, tolerant, and sensitive when dealing with indigenous clients.

Despite La Agencia's relative silence about the historical and structural factors that inform the current cultural formations of indigenous migrants and those who seek to help them, the social and racial inequalities between those who provide services and those who receive them are often revealed during the question-and-answer period of the training. As Luz and Jorge explained to me, and as I also witnessed on multiple occasions, service providers often wondered aloud why *they* should change *their* behavior to accommodate indigenous migrants who have "made the choice" to come to the United States. The inference was that indigenous migrants should be the ones who must change their behavior to assimilate to U.S. culture.

These kinds of "blame the victim" comments reflect a broader sentiment about immigrants and immigration illuminated by the Greenfield case, and they frame immigration as an individual decision rather than an effect of unjust policies and economic systems. Such comments tie the audience's tolerance of cultural difference and their contingent "improvement in manners" to the demand that immigrants take personal responsibility for having to migrate and for all of the things that happen to them once they do. This outcome is the exact opposite of what the cultural sensitivity training hopes to achieve, but as Luz informed me, "It happens all the time." Given that audience members are not made aware of the ways that cultural differences are historically produced, such quid pro quo thinking in which providers will change their attitudes when migrants change their culture is understandable. However, such behavioral differences—like the lack of eye contact or Mexicans saying "*mándame ustéd*" (command me, sir or ma'am) or simply "*mande?*" when asking someone to repeat something—are neither biological nor ontological; they are, instead, an effect of colonial relations. The exclusive focus on cultural difference and migrant vulnerability, accompanied by a demand for cultural accommodation and sensitivity, does not sit well with some nonprofit workers who themselves are living precarious lives and wondering who will accommodate or tolerate them if they transgress the laws and norms of society.

If La Agencia's presentation *did* discuss the historical and political forces informing indigenous migration, audience members would be aware that in many cases the so-called choice so often (and easily) mentioned in immigration debates is a choice between life and death for the migrant and the migrant's family, not necessarily a reflection of their burning desire to embrace and experience U.S. culture. As it stands, La Agencia presents Oaxacan culture without discussing its origins. At the same time, the cultural sensitivity presentation does not engage values in the U.S. health, family, legal, or social systems. The two systems are discussed as if they are simply "different," implying that they are equal and reflecting an apolitical multiculturalism that, as Mignolo explains, "concede[s] 'culture' while maintaining epistemology."[47] In other words, cultural "difference" is in fact repressed under the guise of attending to it. This naturalizes U.S. systems and their rationalities as the norm, thereby creating Oaxacan values, norms, and culture as deviant. This normal/deviant binary was

evident in the Greenfield case discussed at the outset of the chapter. It is a racialized division worked out on the terrain of culture.

As the cultural sensitivity trainers dissect and define for service providers
the value systems of indigenous Oaxacans, those same providers are not asked
to critically and consciously learn about and reflect on their own value systems,
worldviews, or embodied understandings. This sets up a power dynamic in
which the service providers can maintain their belief that they are normal and
rational because they have cultural institutions grounded in science, law, education, and ultimately civilization on their side. In contrast, Oaxacans are perceived as deviant, backward, traditional, and, ultimately, "different" because
they don't have a lot of education or because they practice alternative medicine.
This power dynamic reflects Foucault's notion of episteme: "The episteme is
the 'apparatus' which makes possible the separation not of the true from the
false, but of what may from what may not be characterized as scientific."[48] Those
perceived as lacking "scientificity" or scientific knowledge are also seen to lack
civilization.

The cultural sensitivity training fails to challenge service providers to
rethink and reshape their own epistemological and ontological formations, their
ways of being and knowing, even as it proposes that there are other ways of
being human. But that is not its only effect. It also gives service providers added
power because now they "know" the indigenous "other" and can use this knowledge to help the poor Oaxacans whose superstitious beliefs in *mal de ojo* or
nervios can be relativized and repathologized in terms of depression, anxiety,
or some other seemingly equivalent psychopathology.

The lack of engagement with the cultural differences that make the difference, especially those regarding individual versus collective subjectivity, were
made apparent to me during a discussion at a binational health conference
in Puebla, Mexico, with a professor who teaches at a well-known university in
California. The professor teaches courses about alternative medical systems
and is a therapist working with Mexican migrants, some of whom are indigenous. During our conversation she explained that once we understand what
indigenous Mexicans think they are suffering from, such as *nervios* or *mal de
ojo*, we can use the standard referent for all psychotherapists, the *Diagnostic
and Statistical Manual of Mental Disorders*, to determine what they really have
and develop a treatment plan. In other words, we can compare it to our episte-
mologies and come up with the truth of their pathology. The problem with this
is that psychology, like many of the liberal, Western human sciences, focuses
on the individual as the site of pathology, which, as La Agencia's presentation
discusses, is contrary to the perspective of indigenous Oaxacans. Further, this

individualized and individualizing lens neglects the larger historical and social factors that inform health conditions, such as *nervios*, in migrant populations.

The imbalance of power between service providers and those they are trained to be sensitive about is exacerbated by the fact that service providers can and easily do change jobs, taking the cultural knowledge they have gained with them, just as they would take knowledge they acquire from a museum or a vacation to an "exotic" land. This knowledge translates into economic advantage, as they can claim education and in some cases certification in indigenous cultural competency. Indigenous migrants do not have this luxury, as they can neither abandon their lives nor, in most cases, receive extra compensation for the cultural knowledge they possess. The most they can hope for is continued physical existence, which is increasingly attached to their economic survival.

Because the presentation is set up in terms of "us" and "them," providers, who are themselves often structurally vulnerable, have little opportunity to see how they are similar to indigenous migrants or to identify ways to act in solidarity with them. Such an us versus them binary is evident when the presenters describe the difficulty indigenous people have adapting to their new environment because of social isolation and cultural attachment. The presenters explain, "They stay isolated by choice due to the long history of discrimination and colonization. The isolation goes both ways. They are marginalized and self-marginalizing." This important statement critiques the colonial legacy and its effects on indigenous Oaxacans, couching indigenous behavior in a structural explanation, while also explaining why they might not readily adopt all of the behaviors that service providers would like. It points directly to the causes of structural vulnerability for indigenous Oaxacans and explains their marginalization.

Yet, even as it does this important political work, this statement reinscribes a cultural essentialization that assumes cultural isolation or assimilation are the only two options for indigenous migrants in the United States. The everyday realities, in which migrants interact with actors from diverse race and class backgrounds, including powerful community and civic leaders, challenge the notion that they either fully resist or fully surrender to an American lifestyle. These realities also challenge the notion that culture, whether ours or theirs, is homogeneous and static. Because indigenous ways of being and knowing are produced by and within particular historical, geographic, political, economic, social, and cultural contexts, they are dynamic and evolving. Indeed, critical anthropologists argue that "in a world subjected for centuries to the forces of European capitalism and imperialism, anthropological assumptions about cultural continuity, autonomy and authenticity must be questioned. Much of what appears ancient, integrated, and in need of preservation against the disruptive impact of modern social change is itself recently invented."[49] While many indigenous migrants do live in situations of extreme vulnerability, and the cultural politics in the United States does put them at a significant disadvantage, they are not powerless and often find ways to engage strategically with the dominant system while defining themselves as indigenous. The cultural sensitivity workshops can be understood as one way of doing this.

Conclusion: Teaching Structural Competency

Through an analysis of La Agencia's cultural sensitivity training this chapter has sought to illuminate the cultural politics at work when indigenous migrants teach service providers to be more sensitive, empathetic, and tolerant. One of the key findings is that there are many more cultures at work in La Agencia's trainings than just "indigenous Oaxacan culture." For instance, the dominant cultural orientations and assumptions of the service providers who attend the workshops shape the narratives that La Agencia has to work against—indeed, they are the reason for the workshops in the first place—but they also shape what can and cannot be said about indigenous culture within the cultural sensitivity workshops themselves.

La Agencia's attempts to teach service providers about Oaxacan indigenous culture recuperate subjugated knowledges and promote ideas about what it means to be indigenous that differs from the highly publicized and stigmatizing representations discussed earlier. Through their presentation, La Agencia staff show that there is more than one way to live and to be in the world. In so doing, they are inviting their audience to reflect on an "other" way of being human—an indigenous way of thinking and living in the world—that has been shaped by traditions that span millennia. In a largely anti-immigrant context, and working against centuries of colonialism and decades of conservative legislation that seeks to undermine affirmative action, multiculturalism, and the social benefits conferred by the welfare state, La Agencia staff are boldly reconstructing civic space to incorporate indigenous peoples as important social actors who claim both rights and recognition. Thus, their cultural training aims to mitigate social inequity by replacing negative cultural images and stereotypes with new representations, not only of what it means to be indigenous but of what it means to be human.

In so doing, however, La Agencia's strategies for educating the community complicate, and possibly undermine, their antiracism struggles. This is the case because, first and foremost, not everything that distinguishes indigenous from nonindigenous peoples has to do with indigenous culture. The narrative at the outset of this chapter, as well as the discussion of structural vulnerability in chapter 2, shows that myriad structural forces produce the differences so easily attributed exclusively to indigenous culture. Additionally, there is not one Oaxacan indigenous culture. With over sixty-eight languages and 364 registered dialects spoken across thirty-two states in Mexico, and seventeen different languages spoken in Oaxaca alone, it is impossible to homogenize the lived realities of indigenous Mexicans and to subsume them all under the umbrella of "Oaxacan culture," as La Agencia's training does.

Cultures are dynamic, and they reflect the changing meanings, ideas, and perceptions of their practitioners. As indigenous Mexicans migrate to the United States, their cultures change, as do their self-understandings. For example, at least one of the promotoras I worked with reported having a greater sense of her indigenous language and community once she came to the United States. Her experience is not unique insofar as La Agencia and BIRM help indigenous migrants in California learn about and practice indigenous cultural traditions, including language, music, dance, and food. Their efforts at turning negative ascription into positive affirmation are part of the cultural shift they hope to bring about within the indigenous migrant community so that indigenous Oaxacans will adopt these practices and be proud of their identities, languages, and heritage. In their cultural sensitivity training La Agencia employees do not highlight the diverse forces that influence indigenous cultures, and they spend little time explaining the ways that indigenous migrants are both changed by and themselves changing the communities they move into. Because of this, they risk reinforcing a stereotypical and atavistic understanding of indigenous culture.

If they were to make their cultural sensitivity trainings more nuanced, however, they would risk jeopardizing the funding and support of their audience members. Staff members are hesitant to point out, for example, that there is a need for social services because of unjust trade policies with Mexico, xenophobic immigration policies in the United States, historic anti-indigenous racism and genocide, and a long-standing belief that farmworkers, domestics, and service workers—all sectors where indigenous migrants work—don't deserve a living wage. They also avoid saying that a Christian view of salvation that has posited indigenous peoples as uncivilized and in need of saving shapes how indigenous populations are perceived by nonindigenous peoples.[50] In other words, if they were to flip the approach in the trainings by pointing out how the cultural orientations and interpretive frameworks of nonindigenous people were also to blame for the "culture clashes" described at the outset of this chapter, then they might anger their audience members whose altruism functions best by ignoring these important facts. Indeed, it is the fear of a racist backlash and the potential to lose vital economic support that ultimately prevents La Agencia from actually doing the more robust antiracism work that they would like to do and that would, ultimately, lead to better health outcomes for indigenous people.

La Agencia's conundrum is not unusual: one of the ways that cultural politics gets shaped is through racism. Jordan and Weedon explain, "Racism is a cultural and institutional phenomenon, not fundamentally a matter of individual psychology, not of 'racists' or 'prejudiced individuals.' It is deeply ingrained within the dominant social structures and signification systems of contemporary Western societies."[51] Because dominant systems in the United States, including cultural institutions, were founded on racism, it is difficult for people raised within the U.S. context to see that their viewpoints are both shaped by and reflect this structural racism. It is also difficult for them to see how structural racism shapes the behaviors and cultures of racialized groups.

Referring specifically to the Black experience, but making a broader point about the power of representational discourse for shaping self-understanding, cultural theorist Stuart Hall illuminates the stakes of racism for racialized populations: "They had the power to make us see and experience ourselves as 'Other.' Every regime of representation is a regime of power formed, as Foucault reminds us, by the fatal couplet 'power/knowledge.' But this kind of knowledge is internal not external. It is one thing to position a subject or set of peoples as Other in a dominant discourse. It is quite another thing to subject them to that 'knowledge,' not only as a matter of imposed will and domination, by the power of inner compulsion and subjective conformation to the norm."[52] As a cultural phenomenon, racism causes racialized populations to interrogate their own identities in a continual search to find the reasons they are being discriminated against. It also demands that those same populations continually account for their social, cultural, and phenotypical differences from the dominant group. This is the challenge that La Agencia confronts. In the end, they must offer a cultural explanation to service providers that rides a fine line between cultural affirmation and cultural essentialization. They are compelled to describe and explain themselves to nonindigenous people because the consequences of cultural misunderstandings can be severe, but these descriptions are based on what they think the audience is ready and able to hear and understand.

Even if they fail to fully promote an antiracist politics, however, La Agencia's efforts to promote cultural sensitivity should be understood as a process that opens up space for "other" ways of being and knowing to enter—ways that are considered by indigenous Oaxacans and La Agencia staff to represent a cultural formation that, for political reasons, they wish to invoke as "authentic," even as they recognize that their use of cultural essentialism is both strategic and pragmatic. Given the forces aligned with and validated by dominant cultural representations and ideas, however, La Agencia's pedagogical task is daunting for its employees and complicated for those who, in good faith, are trying to understand what it means to be sensitive to such a diverse and multifaceted population. Until or unless nonindigenous service providers understand that their own cultural presuppositions prevent them from fully understanding the lifeworlds being described by La Agencia and prevent La Agencia from fully describing the ways that those lifeworlds are shaped by racially inflected cultural politics on the one hand, and structural violence on the other, both sides will continue to struggle for understanding.

Following Gayatri Spivak's famous question on whether the subaltern can speak, this leads us to ask whether the subaltern can be heard within the contemporary cultural politics in the United States. Can indigenous Oaxacans be truly audible or intelligible within the static pedagogies of cultural competency? Because of the failures of these pedagogies, critical health scholars have begun promoting structural rather than cultural competency. These scholars contend that locating approaches to racial diversity solely in the attitudes of service providers ignores "the biological, socioeconomic, and racial impacts of upstream decisions on structural factors such as expanding health and wealth disparities."[53] A structurally competent approach theorizes power, especially how power shapes culture, and it critiques systems of oppression, such as racism, sexism, ageism, heterosexism, and ableism.[54] A structurally competent approach also unearths whiteness as the default standard against which all populations are measured, not only in terms of their skin color but also in terms of their attributes, orientations, and knowledge systems. Whiteness is not about essentialized notions of race so much as it is about a way of being, acting, and embodying shared sensibilities, knowledge, and language patterns—cultural attributes, if you will—that were formed within the colonial project. For this reason, a structurally competent approach foregrounds racist and colonial histories over cultural essentializations.[55] Given this, critical health scholars argue that we should jettison cultural competence and instead foster a self-reflexive grappling with racism and colonialism. To continue the status quo is to eliminate the native *as native* under the guise of cultural competency.

Of course, for nonprofits like La Agencia that depend on both grant funding and the continued altruism of service providers, adopting a structurally competent approach in their sensitivity trainings is easier said than done. As this chapter shows, structures rooted in powerful cultural politics that themselves are shaped in racist and colonial histories inform what can be said publicly by indigenous speakers and shape the ways that sensitivity and tolerance can be taught to nonindigenous audiences. Acutely aware of their subjection to the whims of funders and the goodwill of service providers, La Agencia staff actively work to keep good relationships by avoiding controversial programming. In so doing, their work subtly affirms a form of new racism by using culturalist language to frame social and structural difference. Given their constraints, however, it can hardly be otherwise.

This does not mean that their cultural trainings foreclose all possibility of achieving political rights and recognition, however. The work of anthropologist Charles Hale is instructive in this regard. Hale argues that there may be no other way for indigenous groups, and the researchers who seek to help them, to conduct business than to employ the tools and resources that have oppressed indigenous peoples.[56] This strategy, utilized by the Garífuna in their struggle for land rights in Honduras, is informed by the following logic: "Oppressed peoples, in the vast majority of cases, have no alternative but to wage struggles for rights and redress using the language, legal and political tools, and even the funding of their oppressors. They regularly engage in subversion, imbue the dominant with alternative meanings, find room for maneuver, and in so doing, bring about consequences that are quite different than the ones that the dominant actors have in mind."[57] La Agencia has, indeed, found room to maneuver in recent years. In keeping with their creative and pragmatic approaches, they have found several ways to work around the constraints on what they can say and do in their trainings. One of those work-arounds, as illustrated in this chapter, is to collaborate with critical scholars who can publicly discuss controversial dynamics without fear of retribution. Indeed, La Agencia has working relationships with scholars and activists, many of them indigenous, throughout the hemisphere who can and do theorize contemporary power relations between indigenous and nonindigenous communities, and who channel their energies toward illuminating injustice against indigenous peoples.

La Agencia has also begun charging service providers and others who want to access their expertise about indigeneity. Charging for interpretation services, language workshops, cultural competency trainings, and classes on indigenous cultural traditions like cooking or dance gives La Agencia more financial autonomy and thus more freedom with the rest of their programming. This allows them to talk about indigenous identity in the ways they want and also to reimagine, represent, and even remake indigenous culture in new ways, foregrounding its richness, complexity, and beauty while undermining tropes of backwardness and lack of civilization.

Chapter 6

La Lucha Sigue

Migrant Activism and the Ongoing Struggle to Promote Indigenous Health

It is freezing. Literally. It's only February, but the winter of 2007 has been harsh and all of the crops in central California have frozen. There is no work, no money, and soon to be no food for farmworker families. An elderly Mixtec man entered La Agencia's small office on the central coast looking for help. For two weeks all he had eaten were the tomatoes he had stored in his freezer since summer, and they were almost gone. Apologetic, the *promotoras* (community health workers) explained that they couldn't help him because the food bank had run out of food, the Salvation Army had run out of grocery vouchers, and there was nowhere else to send him. Holding his soiled white cowboy hat in one hand and pushing the glass door open with the other, he walked out into the dreary afternoon, shaking his head in dismay.

A few minutes later an elderly Mixtec woman came in. She was upset because they had shut off her power for not paying her bill. Alicia, the Mixtec promotora called the power company to ask if they could work out a payment plan for the unemployed woman, but the power company wouldn't discuss the account because she was not the account holder. Alicia explained that the customer could not speak Spanish or English. The representative on the other end of the line would not budge, however. If the account holder wanted to discuss her situation, she would have to come to the nearest office, over twenty miles away, with an ID card. When Alicia conveyed this information to the woman in Mixtec she responded that she didn't have transportation to get there and that, because her husband was working out of state, she didn't have anyone to interpret for her. It was also not clear that she had an ID to show, even if she could get there. Alicia promised to take her the next day to see if they could sort things out.

That night a local community organizer held a meeting for the indigenous migrant community. Because it was winter many of the local men had gone to other parts of the state and country to work. It was, therefore, mostly women with children in strollers and elderly people who showed up to the meeting room behind a local church. They had come with the promise of information about where they could get help with their rent, electricity bills, and, most importantly, food. The organizer was a trusted source of information and known to just about everyone who had come out. The room was buzzing as people greeted their friends, shared their stories, and expressed their hopes. As the meeting began, however, it was quickly apparent that the only resources available were for those who had legal documents to be in the United States. Echoing what the promotoras had told everyone who had come into the office earlier that day, all of the local resources for undocumented migrant farmworkers had run out. There was nothing anyone could offer. Disappointed, and in relative silence except for a few crying babies, the scores of people who had walked many blocks in the cold to attend the meeting, trickled back out into the darkness.

The next day as we drove the elderly Mixtec woman to the power company, the two promotoras railed against the community organizer. They were angry at him for getting people's hopes up, for making them come out in freezing weather for nothing, and then for making them feel bad because they didn't have legal status in the United States. "He should have known better," Berta fumed. "He just wanted to make it seem like he was doing something," Alicia charged. I agreed that he should have known that those who would attend the meeting would likely not qualify for the resources he was offering. At the same time, I wondered what would happen if, instead of turning their anger on him, they directed it at the political, economic, and social systems that rendered migrant workers unqualified for the resources needed to ensure that both their basic human needs and their human rights were met.

Through an examination of La Agencia's Indigenous Health Project, *Embodied Politics* set out to explore the influential force of public health promotion in the lives of indigenous Oaxacans at the height of their out-migration to California. Working from the premise that neither indigenous cultures nor health cultures are static, there were two questions driving this book: First, in what ways were indigenous cultures entangled with, influenced by, or coproduced in relation to a "culture of health" in the United States during the period under study? Second, what were the effects of these entanglements on indigenous Mexican migrants? In asking these questions I expected that I would discover political and practical ways of supporting activist efforts to promote indigenous health practices. Instead, I discovered that the entanglements between indigeneity and health were more complicated than I had imagined. Despite all of health promotion's promises about community empowerment and cultural competency, not only was there not a smooth integration of indigenous culture into health promotion programs, there were competing agendas at work within the Indigenous Health Project (IHP). The tensions were informed by the promotion of several non-health-related phenomena, including cultural maintenance versus cultural change, freedom versus subjection, and tradition versus novelty.

These tensions set up a core paradox in which the health promotion workshops utilized culturally and linguistically competent methods to encourage indigenous migrants to adopt neoliberal ways of being, including taking individual responsibility for their health in the United States. Because of structural barriers, however, the program participants were often prevented from actually taking control of their health. The upshot of this paradox is that by focusing on individual lifestyle and behavior change, the IHP was teaching its program participants to adapt their behaviors and their lifestyles to often inaccessible and inhumane structures. What might have had a more positive influence on indigenous health and flourishing, however, would have been to teach people, program participants, and service providers alike to understand and work toward changing those structures instead. Once I identified this paradox, I sought to explore how the program participants and staff of the IHP negotiated it.

The situation that many indigenous migrants found themselves in during the 2007 freeze is illustrative of the kinds of dynamics that the paradox engenders. In the midst of that cold winter, indigenous migrants actively sought out the help of the promotoras; they rationed their food almost to starvation; they tried to apply for rental, food, and utility assistance; they gathered information at a community meeting; and they attempted to do everything in their power to take individual responsibility for their diet, housing conditions, bills, and family needs. Yet, the legal, economic, political, and social structures they encountered prevented them from actually being able to improve their situations. No matter how willing they were to become active health citizens, availing themselves of every opportunity to insure and ensure their health, they could neither access nor change the systems that denied them health and housing benefits nor could they control the economic structures that failed to pay them a living wage or to provide them unemployment assistance so that they could cover their basic housing and food costs. No matter how willing the promotoras were to help them, they also could not change the inaccessible structures that they and their program participants encountered. As the foregoing examples show, the combination of culturally and linguistically competent support services offered through the IHP and the individual incentive of its program participants can only go so far if those efforts are not met with equally accessible and supportive systems and structures.

La Agencia did not intend to contribute to this paradoxical dynamic. In response to the structural violence that indigenous Oaxacans encountered in both Mexico and the United States, the indigenous activists that formed La Agencia envisioned the IHP as a way to promote indigenous cultural maintenance and self-determination alongside indigenous health. Nevertheless, La Agencia's founding corresponded with an increased philanthropic focus on health promotion in the United States, one that entailed a shift in the responsibility for population health from the state to individuals and a coincident demand for numerical accountability and transparency on behalf of those individuals. As health promotion became the philanthropic "flavor of the month," indigenous migrants increasingly drew upon it as both a conceptual and an economic resource to meet their needs and to become empowered as indigenous subjects in the United States. Although this model started out as a way to protect the health of everyone, especially the world's poor, with time it ended up as a way to enroll communities in managing their own health and "owning" the responsibility for the outcomes that ensued. In other words, it went from "health for all" to "all for health." Because of the strong policy influence of neoliberalism in the science, politics, and economics of health promotion, the messages that participants in the IHP received and the imperatives that the program staff worked under strongly reflected the values that neoliberalism promotes, including prudent and calculative rationalities, economic competition, quantitative accountability, and an overwhelming sense of individual responsibility.

On the surface, La Agencia's use of health promotion to also promote indigenous culture resonates strongly with the social justice aspect of health that many in the public health field, including researchers, philanthropists, and activists, ascribe to. By affirming the biological and cultural existence of indigenous peoples, health promotion functions as a powerful activist tool in a broader repertoire of civic technologies. Through the promotion of indigenous health, La Agencia staff members and their program participants have been able to access life-sustaining resources, interface with political leaders, navigate complex legal and health care systems, and understand their individual health risks. These factors have contributed to a stronger sense of confidence for the program participants of the IHP who feel that they have a powerful institution, a culturally competent staff, and vital health information to support them in moments of uncertainty or precarity. At the same time, however, the information the health workshops provided has also contributed to a growing sense of anxiety for some of the program participants, making them feel that they are perpetually at risk. Further, in shaping indigenous self-understandings the health workshops also subtly conduct the conduct of program participants by teaching them what and how to think about their bodies, what aspects of their health to value, and how to behave in the United States according to dominant norms—norms that are in tension with their cultural maintenance efforts.

The IHP is successful at teaching its program participants how to be good, neoliberal health citizens *because* the programs are run by linguistically and culturally competent promotoras, not in spite of this fact. Indigenous Mexicans feel compelled to embrace, if not always practice, the health norms promoted within the IHP because, as the case of Jesus Martinez Galindo discussed in chapter 5 demonstrates, they are often punished when their practices are defined as too different from mainstream society. Indigenous migrants are also compelled by the need for resources and information to navigate their lives in the United States. As Jeronimo once expressed to me when I asked him whether there were things in the health workshops that didn't match up with his culture, "Everything makes sense for life here because people work so hard here and it is different than Mexico."

Reflecting the performative aspects of indigenous identity, culturally and linguistically competent health programs are a way for indigenous migrants to "make sense" of indigenous life, of indigenous bodies, and of indigenous selves in the United States. Armed with the knowledge of how to live healthy lives, they are empowered to engage in self-care and to pursue healthy practices as these are defined within the dominant public health episteme. At the same time, cultural competency pedagogies are a way for nonindigenous practitioners to "make sense" of indigenous Mexican migrants in ways that reproduce uninterrogated differences without ever questioning how those differences were produced in the first place. As I have shown throughout this book, however, both the promotion of indigenous culture to nonindigenous service providers and the promotion of neoliberal health to indigenous program participants are not without contestation and resistance. Convincing both of these groups to adopt the dominant narratives is an ongoing struggle and an objective that we should continue to question.

Implications of the Analysis

There are several implications that follow from my analysis. The first is that a subjectively practiced indigenous culture should not be viewed in opposition to a seemingly neutral and apolitical health science. Health science has a history and a politics to it. As I discussed in chapter 3, although we use the term "health promotion" to describe a phenomenon that involves teaching people how to care for their health, the values, stakes, and methods for conducting the promotion of health have changed across time and space. We, therefore, need to be mindful of what we are promoting when we are promoting health. When we promote health we are also promoting an embodied politics under the guise of scientific neutrality. As Deborah Lupton explains, "It may be argued that the discourses and practices around the promotion of health have been central to constituting the contemporary human body. More so than perhaps any other apparatus or institution, discourses on health and illness serve as routes through which to understand, think and talk about, and live our bodies."[1] Taken together, and in order to understand what is meant by "indigenous health," then, we need to be attentive to the changing science of social science, and to the dynamic natures of both health and indigeneity.

While indigenous peoples have a number of health and medical repertoires that they draw from to care for their health, they are pragmatic about which ones they use. Anthropologist Bonnie Bade has used the term "transmedicalization" to describe this practice whereby indigenous women and their families move between distinct health care systems (with differing values, methods, languages, behaviors, and schedules) and along diverse pathways to attend to their medical needs in the United States. She explains, "The movement implied by the word 'trans' refers not only to the migrant nature of the Mixtec lifestyle but also to the complex systems—social, political, and economic—that Mixtec families navigate to achieve health care."[2] Bade notes that while indigenous families, like anyone else, want full health care coverage, the reality in the United States is that for undocumented families clinical care is limited; thus they must negotiate their health with the tools at their disposal. Health promotion has been a ready tool for them.

Related to this is the idea that cultures are not always or ever simply a feature of an individual population. Institutions, disciplines, and domains, like health, have cultures. These cultures are lived and practiced in a variety of ways, and they are always evolving in relation to broader social, political, historical, scientific, technological, and economic phenomena. This makes it very difficult to become "competent" about any one of them, let alone cultures that are practiced by a mobile, dynamic, multilingual, multiethnic population like indigenous Mexican migrants. Indigenous peoples and the institutions they develop are complex, and their cultures are polyvalent. Just as they negotiate multiple medical repertoires, they also juggle a variety of contemporary political, economic, social, cultural, and linguistic practices at the same time that they maintain and reproduce their ancestral systems as distinctive peoples and communities. Indigenous Mexican migrants are resilient and pragmatic; as such they find ways to survive in uncertain and hostile conditions.

This leads to a third point. Not everything that distinguishes indigenous people from nonindigenous people has to do with "their" culture. Structural forces, such as immigration policy, health care markets, trade policies, histories of colonization, and racism, aided by knowledge systems and economic priorities, produce, solidify, and naturalize the differences that we see between indigenous and nonindigenous groups. Importantly, visible cultural markers of difference mask the similarities between and within social groups. For example, by focusing on seemingly natural and static differences we fail to see that many of us are similarly positioned with regard to the demands of and inequities generated by neoliberal capitalism. Most of us are losing ground, albeit at different rates and in different ways, in a system of growing economic inequity and uncertainty. In addition, all of us are implicated by and within racial, gender, sexual, and scientific hierarchies that bestow varying levels of rights, recognition, privilege, and vulnerability.

We can lose sight of the ways that these social, political, and economic systems work in each of our lives and on each of our bodies when we focus too much on our differences. Rather than focusing on cultural difference, one of the takeaway points from my analysis, then, is that instead of trying to become competent about the cultural "other," we should instead work to recognize and understand our structural similarities. We should become structurally competent. Physician and sociologist Jonathan Metzl makes the case for structural competency, arguing that, "at a time when income disparities grow, and notions of health become increasingly politicized, we need new narratives that expertly diagnose how structures and institutions oppress certain persons for the betterment of others, and that methodically demonstrate how these structures and institutions are not timeless monoliths but instead social formations constructed as the result of specific decisions made at particular points in time."[3] Learning to identify and explain the relationship between structural power and embodied outcomes would provide a foundation for engaging in the collective work of creating structures that will truly ensure health for all. Indeed, teaching self-responsibility for health, even in culturally competent ways, is no substitute for developing social, political, and economic structures that truly value health and that make it possible for everyone to live a healthy life.

A final implication of my analysis is that freedom and control are related phenomena. One of the broader points of *Embodied Politics* is that indigenous culture is an important mechanism through which social justice is fomented. It

is, at the same time, an important mechanism through which indigenous subjection occurs. These two processes are not separate. For, even as it promotes
freedom from the historical forces that have disparaged indigenous cultures and
exterminated indigenous peoples, the IHP simultaneously works to regulate the
behaviors, thoughts, and actions of indigenous groups so that they align more
closely with the dominant norms and values in U.S. society. Contrary to the idea
that indigenous health promotion is emancipatory, then, the cultural mecha-
nisms for empowering indigenous migrants to become healthy citizen subjects
are normalizing, regulating, and subjectifying. Thus, both the promotion of
indigenous identity and the promotion of indigenous health operate as productive political technologies bringing the ideals and aspirations of indigenous
migrants into alignment with neoliberal social norms, and the varied institutions that uphold them.

    Insofar as much of the struggle for indigenous autonomy and sovereignty
in Mexico has been against the encroachment of neoliberal policies and practices in their communities, the idea that indigenous migrants are adopting neoliberal values to survive in the United States has implications for what it means
to be indigenous and what it means to promote indigenous health. This generates important questions about what an activist health politics could or should
look like when promoting indigenous health is increasingly synonymous with
promoting neoliberal subjectivity and when community empowerment and
community control are two sides of the same coin. While I don't have a clear
answer to this, one place to start is by examining the values that health itself is
promoting, rather than promoting health as if it were neutral and apolitical. This
book has offered some material for reflection on that matter.

From Cultural Competency to Structural Competency

Much of what I have written in this book is driven by my dissatisfaction with
the uses of culture in health care, particularly with attempts to teach practitioners to be culturally competent. My discontent stems from what I have come to
see as the ahistorical givenness of culture within cultural trainings, particularly
how these trainings begin with the fact of difference rather than an exploration
of how difference is constituted. Within both the mainstream literature and
practices of cultural competence, it seems that culture "just happens" devoid of
power or context. It also appears that culture only "happens" to marginalized
groups whose cultural ways of being and knowing are framed as entrenched and
permanent. By contrast, dominant groups function, on the one hand, as if they
have a culture of no culture, and on the other hand, by learning the culture of

the other (becoming competent) in order to succeed in understanding or assimilating them.[4]

The assumption in much of the literature is that migrants will assimilate to what is loosely referred to as U.S. culture, a nebulous term that obscures more than it explains. The belief that cultural evolution is unidirectional fails to grapple with the ways that unmarked white, middle-class U.S. citizens are also changing their cultural practices in relation to new waves of migrants, however. An oversimplified yet clear example of this cultural shift is exemplified in the fact that salsa is outselling ketchup in the United States, as anthropologist Arlene Davila has pointed out.[5] It also fails to grapple with the uneven power dynamic at work in such cultural assumptions. Seth Holmes is instructive in this regard. He argues that many immigrant health researchers blame poor health outcomes on a lack of culture or assimilation, utilizing poorly defined constructs like "religiosity" or "machismo" as a proxy for immigrant culture. Regardless of the specifics, he writes, "These frameworks include troubling assumptions of a unidirectional move from a 'traditional' culture to a culture of the assumed modern, unmarked white American middle class."[6] The ways that marked cultural others are produced in relation to unmarked cultureless selves remain uninterrogated in such assumptions.

Not only does cultural competency too frequently contribute to subtle forms of new racism, the uses of culture in health research often obscure the intersectional structural forces that influence health outcomes.[7] For example, in their article on culture as the missing link in health research, Marjorie Kagawa Singer and her colleagues argue that culture is often proposed as an explanatory variable for difference in health outcomes, yet little work explicates the precise cultural processes involved. Instead, "nominal proxy cultural "markers" reflect truncated, static conceptualizations that hamper our ability to understand the actual forces informing health behavior at the individual, group or institutional levels of society, including health care itself."[8] Given this, the authors suggest that representations of cultural practices or identities have questionable external validity and are of little use in either improving equity in the health status of diverse populations or moving the science of health forward.[9]

Anthropologists, whose work historically traffics in the domain of culture, argue that in order to overcome the static and stereotypical uses of culture in health care we must document the social processes by which what is uncontested, that is, what is perceived as not cultural, is produced and reproduced.[10] This includes revealing competing discourses and practices within situations characterized by the unequal distribution of power and pointing to the

structures that produce and reproduce them. As Holmes writes, "Health researchers must move beyond such apolitical analyses of health as based only in individual and cultural behaviors and instead begin to recognize and point out
the unequal social, economic, and political structures that produce poor health
outcomes in the first place."[11]

Understanding how differences in wealth, in social standing, in culture, and
in health outcomes are produced across specific times and particular spaces
requires structural, not cultural, competency. As critical health scholars have
argued, cultural competency may actually distract providers' attention from
more relevant targets of intervention, like the structural forces that overdeter-
mine their life circumstances and health behaviors.[12] In a context of structural
inequity, very little about the social status, economic position, or negative health
outcomes of indigenous Mexican migrants has to do with what their cultural
traditions have taught them, about what languages they speak, what they wear,
or what they eat. It is not that indigenous cultures and languages are irrelevant,
in fact they have significant health-protective factors. It is rather that when it
comes to the morbidity and mortality of this population, structural factors play
an outsized role. While structural competency will not solve all of the barriers
to good health that indigenous Mexican migrants confront, it will keep the origins of those problems, rather than the behaviors of those who experience them,
front and center in the discussion.

I recognize that, in light of the significant contributions of poststructural-
ism and the turn to more dynamic explanatory frameworks in the social
sciences, a focus on structures may seem out of date, too static, or to lack a
nuanced analysis of the relationship between people and the worlds they
inhabit. While *Embodied Politics* has used both structural and poststructural
theories to make its arguments, it has particularly pushed for a return to the
study of structures in health outcomes for a reason. Calling attention to the role
that structural forces, especially neoliberal capitalism, play in the health and
well-being of poor and indigenous populations builds on a long tradition of critical health scholarship produced by those working in and from Latin America.[13] It also builds on the emerging work of critical scholars working at the
intersection of the social sciences and biomedicine.[14]

The most important reason for focusing on neoliberal capitalism, however,
is to complicate many of the socioecological models in public health that
position public policy, culture, or general socioeconomic, cultural, and environmental conditions as the factors that shape all other aspects of population,
community, or individual health and wellness. In many of the nested models
that public health scholars develop to explain or envision the social determi-

nants of health, these more general factors are placed on the periphery, in the broadest bubble, to explain their influence on the next layer down. But the question that I have, and which this book has sought to illuminate, is what is shaping those political, cultural, socioeconomic, and environmental conditions. My focus on neoliberalism seeks to complicate those public health models by showing how the values and imperatives of neoliberalism are not only one among many peripheral social determinants of health, but are themselves determining forces in all the social determinants of health at every level of the multilayered model. That said, what neoliberalism looks like, how it is practiced, and how it gets negotiated at each of the different levels are empirical questions that should continue to be asked.

The Evolution of Indigenous Activism

What I have written in this book is but a snapshot of the ongoing activist practices of indigenous Mexican migrants in California. Much has changed in terms of these practices since I conducted the original research. One of the most significant changes is that La Agencia has enacted a number of personnel changes that reflect their long-standing goals of cultivating female leadership and youth activism. For example, whereas the organization was founded and historically run by men, it is currently run by two women. Lillia, a Zapotec woman who is the current executive director, was a youth organizer that came up through the organization's youth leadership program, went on to get her doctorate, and then came back to lead the agency. Alejandra, a Mixtec woman who has been involved with La Agencia since its inception, is a skilled community organizer who excels at popular education. As the program director, she organizes community workshops on a variety of issues related to social justice, including the importance of being counted in the census, the right to have an interpreter, and the need for immigration reform. Together, these two women have shifted the direction of the organization from its earlier focus on service provision to a focus on sustainable structural change.

This new direction was evident in a conversation I had with Lillia over Zoom in spring 2021. During our call she shared one of her main challenges as the incoming executive director, "I'm afraid of always being service-based" because, as she lamented, "[service] navigation does not work!" Instead of always responding to problems, she argued, "We need to think about how to address things in a more structural way." Lillia's words clearly illustrate the paradox that informed earlier iterations of La Agencia's programs in which teaching newly arriving migrants to eat better, exercise, and go to the doctor did not change the circumstances that made them sick in the first place. Her words also illustrate the ways that a change in organizational leadership is leading to a change in organizational focus. For Lillia, it feels urgent that she work to change systems and structures, otherwise she worries about getting caught in an endless rut of service provision, teaching people how to navigate the existing, mostly inaccessible, systems and to embrace "healthier" lifestyles, without ever really disrupting the causes of their suffering. As she told me, "You can't force people to navigate structures if you are not changing structures."

My Zoom call with Lillia reminded me of a presentation given by Rishi Manchada, a medical doctor, the founder of HealthBegins and the author of *The Upstream Doctors: Medical Innovators Track Sickness to Its Source*.[15] In the basement of a small community clinic in Galveston, Texas, Dr. Manchada explained the logic of "upstreamism" by reciting a parable to a group of my medical school colleagues and students. In this parable three friends are standing on the shore of a river when they begin to see a child floating by in the water and headed for a waterfall. The first child is followed by many more. Two of the friends rush in to pull the children out, trying to save them from drowning. The third friend, the upstreamist, heads upriver to find out who is throwing the children in the river in the first place. Likening this parable to the way that medicine works—intervening when there's a problem but never getting to the social, political, or economic root of the problem in order to stop it from happening in the first place—Dr. Manchada advocated that health professionals move upstream in both their thinking and their practice. Lillia's concern for structural change resonated with Manchada's focus on upstreamism.

In addition to invoking a kind of upstreamist thinking in health, Lillia's leadership approach reflects several broader dynamics shaping contemporary indigenous migrant activism. One of these has to do with the fact that many of the early supporters and allies of La Agencia have gone on to join state-level agencies and boards, like the Agricultural Labor Relations Board, where they are able to educate their peers about indigenous Mexican migrants and to influence state-level labor policies. Because of these high-level roles, the onus for educating policymakers or for changing the political and economic status quo no longer falls exclusively on the shoulders of newly arriving and highly vulnerable indigenous migrants, nor do these activities rely on the magnanimity, whims, and permission of philanthropic organizations. Indigenous migrants, their adult children, and their advocates literally now have a seat at the table. Lillia elaborated on how being raised in the United States has made her think and act differently than first-generation migrants. Comparing herself to her forebears, she said that she feels a sense of entitlement to her rights that they did not feel. "They were so humble and willing to accept things. They had that migrant mentality. I don't have that," she tells me, "probably because I grew up here."

The sense of self-efficacy that Lillia feels is related to another broad dynamic. Due to the hard work and perseverance of earlier generations, there is now a growing cadre of well-educated indigenous scholars and activists who know their rights and, like Lillia, feel entitled to them. These college graduates, who hold bachelor's, master's, and doctoral degrees, are increasingly called upon to share their expertise with important power brokers across diverse sectors, including the agricultural industry, academia, and law enforcement. Rather than seeking out powerful institutions and actors to ask for their support and cultural understanding, indigenous activists and their allies are themselves being sought out for their knowledge and expertise and, as a result, are shaping the structures that used to be both inaccessible to and ignorant of them.

I was able to learn more about the influential roles that indigenous scholars and activists are playing in California during a brief visit I took to Los Angeles in fall 2019. I went to L.A. because I had been asked by a prominent journal in Latinx studies to review a scholarly article that was using a cultural competency framework to evaluate and revise labor-related educational materials for California farmworkers. Explicitly addressing my critiques of cultural competency, the article had drawn on a piece that I had published in the same journal a few years earlier. As I reviewed the article two things occurred to me. First, although the authors said they were using a cultural competency framework, once I read their methodology I saw that they were actually using structural not cultural competency to conduct their evaluation of the educational materials. Second, I realized that across the time and distance, through scholarly publications, the conversation about which methods are best for doing the kind of decolonial, antiracist, social justice work that we are all invested in remains dynamic and ongoing. Just as the meanings of what it means to be indigenous are evolving, so, too, are the methods for developing a transformative activist praxis.

Eager to further the discussion, I contacted one of the article's authors and asked if we could talk. He graciously agreed and coordinated a meeting with himself and a number of L.A.-based activists. A few weeks later I was sitting around a U-shaped table surrounded by indigenous activist-scholars who have dedicated their lives to the dual focus of improving the well-being of indigenous Mexicans and to shattering the stereotypes about them. The primary author of the article was on the speaker phone. We began the conversation by discussing cultural competency and whether it was the best method for communicating the life experiences of indigenous Mexican migrants to nonindigenous service providers. We also talked about the differences between cultural and structural competency. Soon, however, several members of the group grew tired of the "academic talk" and wanted to focus on the real needs of indigenous migrants. These included the need for interpretation in legal, medical, and educational settings; the economic needs of indigenous migrants; and the need to address the racism they experienced at work and in other institutional environments. They wanted to talk about how these things could be addressed, and to share their ongoing efforts.

Two of the women who were present, a powerful mother–daughter team, explained that they had recently made the choice to move away from philanthropic funding and toward crowd-sourced funding. That way they could make all of the decisions about programming themselves. In bypassing the traditional funding routes, they were also able to use and redistribute the funds as they liked without having to respond to the agendas and accountability requirements of philanthropic foundations. Their approach seems to be successful. Through careful fund raising, they were able to raise and redistribute over a million dollars of food and financial aid to indigenous migrants in the Los Angeles area during the first few months of the pandemic. In addition to their direct community work, the women informed me that they had been instrumental in training indigenous interpreters in California. As part of their work to preserve and maintain indigenous languages, they have organized an annual interpreters conference as well as an annual indigenous literature conference.

At the end of my visit to L.A. it occurred to me that, just as my own thinking about how best to support the indigenous community had evolved and changed since the time I first started working with La Agencia, so too had that of the indigenous community. This was exactly the same impression I had when speaking with Lillia over a year later. Leadership training, advocacy, civic engagement, immigration reform, indigenous language acquisition, and interpretation services have all become part of the broader agenda of indigenous organizations and activists throughout California. Unlike the early days, when La Agencia staff were afraid to speak of racism or colonization for fear of jeopardizing their funding, as the indigenous movement has grown and their communities have stabilized and become more educated and integrated into California institutions, they have become more comfortable with demanding that their human, civil, labor, and language rights be respected.

Nevertheless, although many changes have taken place in recent years, unfortunately much has also remained the same with regard to the structural conditions that indigenous Mexican migrants face and in terms of the need to keep informing the public about those conditions. In fact, with the onset of the pandemic, there has been a greater need than ever to understand and intervene in the unjust and inequitable living and working conditions that indigenous Mexicans confront throughout the United States. Many of these conditions, unsurprisingly, continue to be driven by the dual forces of structural racism and neoliberal capitalism.

Conclusion: The More Things Change . . .

In fall 2020, farmworkers throughout the United States were subject to another freeze. This time it was not the climate but politics that produced the chilling effect that reverberated throughout the agricultural worker community. As the COVID-19 pandemic was roiling the United States, disproportionately killing Latinxs, Blacks, and Native Americans, the Department of Labor passed a rule to freeze the wages of agricultural workers holding an H-2A work visa, already some of the lowest-paid workers in the U.S. labor market. The wage freeze would reduce farmworker pay by approximately one dollar an hour and would be in effect until 2023.[16] The rule would not only cost farmworkers an estimated $167.76 million per year in wages across the three years of its implementation, it would also add $1.6 billion in COVID bailout funds to agricultural companies, effectively redistributing wealth from farmworkers to their bosses.[17] The Department of Labor implemented this wealth-redistribution scheme at then president Trump's request. Shortly after it went into effect, the president declared that H-2A visas were essential to the economy and food security of the United States and were therefore a national security priority.[18] Foreign farmworkers, who were declared to be essential both to the U.S. economy and to its national security, had their wages frozen at the same time that they were increasingly exposed to COVID-19. News headlines summarized the implications of this dynamic, "Harvest of Shame," "Hidden Hardship," and the most apt, given what followed, "Worked to Death."[19]

The wage freeze, which was temporarily put on hold by a California judge at the end of December 2020, was only one of many intersecting issues affecting the well-being of indigenous Mexican migrants in California during the pandemic. Because they had been designated as essential workers, farmworkers were expected to show up to work. Indeed, they wanted to work. Yet, this meant that they became infected with COVID-19 at nearly three times the rate of other California residents. A study conducted over five months in the Salinas Valley found that workers who spoke only an indigenous language had higher positivity rates—23 percent—than those who spoke only Spanish (12%), and those who could speak English (4%). The study also found that 57 percent of workers who reported experiencing symptoms and 58 percent who had symptoms and later tested positive had continued working when they had symptoms.[20] As one reporter put it, "A lack of access to testing and protective gear, an aging and consolidated health care system and rampant fear of the Trump administration's strict immigration policies has created ideal conditions for the virus to spread across farmworker camps and small towns."[21]

Yet, even where personal protective equipment, handwashing stations, and testing were available, many low-income laborers were resistant to taking tests because, if they were found to be positive, they lacked the resources or living space to self-quarantine for two weeks. They also feared losing their job or being stigmatized in the workplace, especially if they were the sole breadwinner for their extended family.[22] Thus, close proximity, in the fields, in transportation to and from work, and in crowded living conditions, as well as pervasive fear about losing their jobs, about being labeled a "public charge" if they went to the clinic, and about not being able to feed their families, contributed to the disproportionate and deadly impact of the pandemic on indigenous farmworkers. At a time of significant social, economic, political, and biological vulnerability, indigenous Mexican migrants continued to be squeezed between the needs of the market, their own health needs, and inflammatory xenophobic rhetoric. Because of their legal status, many of them were also unable to access stimulus checks, unemployment benefits, or Social Security. Even though their paychecks are taxed at the same rate as those of U.S. citizens, they were and are denied many of the same benefits and resources that citizens receive.

As scholars, activists, and health philanthropists, we need to continue to fight for the human rights, health, and well-being of indigenous Mexican migrants. This means that we need to simultaneously promote both their cultural and their biological survival. We also urgently need to reform the structures and systems that blame indigenous peoples for their vulnerability and that hold them individually responsible for mitigating the embodied effects of structural violence. The first step in this fight is understanding what they, and we, are up against. Although there is still much to do and say, it is my hope that *Embodied Politics* has contributed in some small way to this ongoing effort.

Acknowledgments

It is a misconception that one individual working tirelessly in an isolated room can produce a book. Indeed, this book is the product of many people working tirelessly over the years and in many rooms to listen, read, support, resist, push, and pull in myriad directions so that these pages could be written. I am indebted to and beyond grateful for them all. At the top of the list are Pat Zavella and Jonathan Fox. Without them, this book would never have been conceptualized or pursued. Their support of my ideas and research has meant more than they may ever know. Ronnie Lipschutz has been an incredible mentor and friend throughout the years. I am truly grateful for all that he has done for me and for his ongoing mentorship. Cindy Bale, Glenda Dixon, Jill Esteras, and Vanita Seth also provided early and much appreciated support.

I owe a special debt of gratitude to the faculty and staff in Latina/Latino Studies at the University of Illinois, Urbana-Champaign, where I spent one year as a Chancellor's Postdoctoral Fellow in Ethnic Studies. Thanks to Laura Castañeda, Alicia Rodriguez, Jonathan Xavier Inda, Isabel Molina-Guzmán, Julie Dowling, Gilberto Rosas, and especially to Edna Viruell-Fuentes, whose light and brilliant scholarship touched us all. I also owe thanks to Sonia Alvarez, Claudia de Lima Costa, Veronia Feliu, Norma Klahn, and Millie Thayer for allowing me to be one of the "translocas."

I am indebted to my friends and interlocutors who helped me better understand indigenous health and migration. These include Rufino Domínguez-Santos, Leoncio Vasquez, Gaspar Rivera-Salgado, Nayamin Martínez-Cossio, Oralia Maceda, Merced Oliveira, Estela Ramírez, Jesus Estrada, Odilia Romero, Janet Martinez, Sarait Martinez, Claudio Hernandez, Centolia Maldonado, Bernardo Bautista Ramírez, Dolores Paris Pombo, and many others. They all generously gave of their time and shared their insights with me. I am very grateful for their contributions to my life and to my research. I am also grateful to the indigenous Mexican communities in the Salinas Valley, the San Joaquin Valley, and Santa Barbara County in California, as well as those in and around Huajuapan de León, Tlaxiaco, and Juxtlahuaca in Oaxaca. Through their participation in focus groups, interviews, and community events, they taught me so much about their lives and experiences. I am especially grateful to Anselmo, a health promoter with the IMSS hospital in Huajuapan de León, for his time and help. The IMSS staff in Mexico City allowed me to photocopy hundreds of pages of health promotion manuals and provided me with their time and materials so that I could learn about the "Mexican model" of health promotion; I appreciate their willingness to help me. I also owe a debt of gratitude to Gordon Hull, Andrea Pitts, and to those who organized and attended my talk at the Center for Professional and Applied Ethics at UNC Charlotte.

I am fortunate to have known and been friends with a number of amazing people over the years who have contributed in some way to moving this project forward. Thanks to Marcos Lopez, Marco Mojica, Pascha Bueno-Hansen, Karen Roller, Elvira Gomez, Sonja Brunner, Gina Castañeda, Debbie Burton, Jason Glenn, Jerome Crowder, Howard Brody, Christine Kovic, Francisco (Pancho) Arguelles, Doug Halvorsen, Jennifer Lawrence, C. L. Bohannon, Emily Satterwhite, Philip Olson, Christine Labuski, Nick Copeland, Daniel Breslau, and especially Matthew Wisnioski, Saul Halfon, and Barbara Allen, whose mentorship have been invaluable. I am eternally grateful to you all for your friendship, guidance, and support. Arlene Macdonald has been the best friend anyone could ask for. Her encouragement, brilliance, laughter, strength, and friendship have sustained me in the good times and the bad. Thanks, also, to the many brilliant graduate students from whom I have learned over the years and especially to those who helped bring this book to fruition. They include Jonathan Banda, HungYin Tsai, Brenda Wilson, Shannon Guillot-Wright, Tarryn Abrahams, Ariel Ludwig, Rachel Pearson, and Erica Fletcher.

I owe a special debt of gratitude to my sister Noelle Iles. Her support of my ambitions and her interest in my research have never wavered. I also want to thank my beautiful children, Jean Baptiste and Sophia, for their endless patience; my mom, Sally Caglia, for all of her love and generous support; and Sherry Zagrodnik. Thank you, Aunt Sherry, for always being in my corner. This book is dedicated to Noelle Iles for always believing in me and to my dear friend Steven Washington, whose untimely passing has made me acutely aware of the life-and-death consequences of racism in our society. Your spirit will live on in my work, always.

I am especially indebted to Seth Holmes and Alicia Gaspar de Alba for careful and generous readings of earlier iterations of this book. I would also like to thank two anonymous reviewers. Many thanks also to my editor at Rutgers, Peter Mickulaus, for his infinite patience and kindness as this book underwent several revisions, and to my developmental editor, Jeremy Rehwaldt, for his careful attention to detail.

Research for this book was made possible by generous grants from UC Mexus and from the University of California Office of the President. I have also received support from the Institute for the Medical Humanities at the University of Texas Medical Branch, as well as the Center for Humanities, the College of Liberal Arts and Human Sciences, and the Department of Science, Technology, and Society at Virginia Tech. In addition, I received an award from the National Institutes Loan Repayment Program for health disparities research. This award allowed me to study the ways that health professionals are taught to understand cultural and linguistic diversity.

Notes

Preface

1. In keeping with the ethical conventions of ethnographic research and according to the institutional review board policies, all names are pseudonyms unless the source of the quote has been published or is publicly available.

1. The Paradoxical Politics of Health Promotion

1. M. Everett, "They Say It Runs in the Family: Diabetes and Inheritance in Oaxaca, Mexico," *Social Science & Medicine* 72, no. 11 (2011): 1776–1783; M. Everett and J. N. Wieland, "Diabetes among Oaxaca's Transnational Population: An Emerging Syndemic," *Annals of Anthropological Practice* 36, no. (2012): 295–311; L. S. Pacheco et al., "Prevalence and Correlates of Diabetes and Metabolic Syndrome in a Rural Indigenous Community in Baja California, Mexico," *BMC Public Health* 18, no. 1 (2018): 1397.

2. J. Hubner, "Hispanic Indians: The New Workforce," *San Jose Mercury News*, August 4, 2001.

3. J. Fox and G. Rivera-Salgado, "Building Civil Society among Indigenous Migrants," in *Indigenous Mexican Migrants in the United States*, ed. Jonathan Fox and Gaspar Rivera-Salgado (La Jolla: Center for U.S.-Mexico Studies and Center for Comparative Immigration Studies, UCSD, 2004), 3.

4. Consejo Nacional de Población, Government of Mexico, https://www.gob.mx/conapo.

5. R. Dominguez Santos, "U.S.-Mexico Binational Indigenous Migration" (paper presented at the meeting of the Executive Board of Hispanics in Philanthropy, Oaxaca de Juarez, Oaxaca, Mexico, January 30, 2006).

6. M. R. Day, "Indigenous Mexican Migrants in California: A Tale of Struggle, Organizing, and Survival," *Indian Country Today*, May 30, 2016.

7. McGuire, S. and Georges, J. (2003) "Undocumentedness and Liminality as Health Variables," *Advances in Nursing Science* 26:3, 185–96.

8. A. Gonzalez-Barrera, "More Mexicans Leaving Than Coming to the U.S.," Pew Research Center, November 19, 2015.

9. Fox and Rivera-Salgado, *Indigenous Mexican Migrants*, 3.

10. See Fox and Rivera-Salgado for estimates on indigenous migrants in California. Exact numbers are difficult to discern because of the mobile nature of the migrant population and the census undercount; see Javier Huizar Murillo and Isidro Cerda, "Indigenous Mexican Migrants in the 2000 U.S. Census," in Fox and Rivera-Salgado, *Indigenous Mexican Migrants*, 279–302; Oaxacalifornian Reporting Team / Equipo de Cronistas Oaxacalifornianos, *Voices of Indigenous Oaxacan Youth in the Central Valley: Creating Our Sense of Belonging in California*, University of California Center for Collaborative Research for an Equitable California, Research Report 1 (UC Santa Cruz, July 2013); R. Mines et al., *California's Indigenous Farmworkers*, final report of the Indigenous Farmworker Study (IFS) to the California Endowment, http://indigenousfarmworkers.org.

11. Fox and Rivera-Salgado, *Indigenous Mexican Migrants*, 11.

12. G. Burchell, "Liberal Government and Techniques of the Self," in *Foucault and Political Reason: Liberalism, Neo-liberalism and Rationalities of Government*, ed. Andrew Barry, Thomas Osborne, and Nikolas Rose (University of Chicago Press, 1996), 19.

13. J. X. Inda, *Targeting Immigrants: Government, Technology, and Ethics* (Hoboken, NJ: John Wiley & Sons, 2006).

14. N. Hiemstra, "Immigrant "Illegality" as Neoliberal Governmentality in Leadville, Colorado," *Antipode* 42, no. 1 (2010): 74–102; J. Bickham Mendez, "Gendered Governmentalities and Neoliberal Logics: Latina, Immigrant Women in Healthcare and Social Services," *Journal of Contemporary Ethnography* 49, no. 4 (2020): 481–506.

15. The idea of a universal humanity is often attributed to this book: J. Vasconcelos, *La Raza Cósmica: Misión de La Raza Iberoamericana* (México, DF: Aguilar, 1996).

16. F. Alvarez, "Interpreters Give Voice to the Indigenous," *Los Angeles Times*, October 11, 2004.

17. M. L. Berk and C. L. Schur, "The Effect of Fear on Access to Care among Undocumented Latino Immigrants," *Journal of Immigrant Health* 3, no. 3 (2001): 151–156.

18. A. Petersen, "Risk, Governance and the New Public Health," in *Foucault: Health and Medicine,* ed. Alan Petersen and Robin Bunton (New York: Routledge, 1997): 189–206; D. Lupton, *The Imperative of Health: Public Health and the Regulated Body* (Thousand Oaks, CA: Sage, 1995); Inda.

19. Personal communication with indigenous activist in California, September 22, 2019.

20. N. Rose, "Molecular Biopolitics, Somatic Ethics and the Spirit of Biocapital." *Social Theory & Health* 5, no. 1 (2007): 3–29; N. Rose, *The Politics of Life Itself: Biomedicine, Power, and Subjectivity in the Twenty-First Century* (Princeton, NJ: Princeton University Press, 2006).

21. K. Bell and J. Green, "On the Perils of Invoking Neoliberalism in Public Health Critique," *Critical Public Health* 26, no. 3 (2016): 239–243.

22. E. Kohl-Arenas, *The Self-Help Myth: How Philanthropy Fails to Alleviate Poverty* (Berkeley: UC Press, 2015), 25.

23. M. L. Pratt, "Arts of the Contact Zone," *Profession* (1991): 33–40, https://www.jstor .org/stable/pdf/25595469?casa_token=ohTUdPayhGEAAAAA:uCiFTSyOp897pHux EV_9icd7KUEOaxbYRzysMasUSxNAPOCbRINn2T7pmOB5GH9pIkWcA4qQll3Qtv OjtpTU-ihKCC5HUEmf-_dJiNI_ASCACBy2lmum.

24. P. Wolfe, "Settler Colonialism and the Elimination of the Native," *Journal of Genocide Research* 8, no. 4 (2006): 387–409.

25. E. Kowal, J. Radin, and J. Reardon, "Indigenous Body Parts, Mutating Temporalities, and the Half-Lives of Postcolonial Technoscience," *Social Studies of Science* 43, no. 4 (2013): 465–483.

26. S. A. Radcliffe, "Geography and Indigeneity II: Critical Geographies of Indigenous Bodily Politics," *Progress in Human Geography* 42, no. 3 (2018): 436–445.

27. J. Ashton and H. Seymour, *The New Public Health*, vol. 1 (Milton Keynes: Open University Press, 1988); Alan Petersen and Deborah Lupton, *The New Public Health: Health and Self in the Age of Risk* (Thousand Oaks, CA: Sage, 1996); I. Kickbusch, "The Contribution of the World Health Organization to a New Public Health and Health Promotion," *American Journal of Public Health* 93, no. 3 (2003): 383–388; Theodore H. Tulchinsky and Elena A. Varavikova, *The New Public Health* (Cambridge, MA: Academic Press, 2014).

28. "The Ottawa Charter for Health Promotion, 1986," World Health Organization, https://www.euro.who.int/__data/assets/pdf_file/0004/129532/Ottawa_Charter.pdf.

29. R. Crawford, "Health as a Meaningful Social Practice," *Health* 10, no. 4 (2006): 402.
30. Crawford, 402.
31. Crawford, 409.
32. Inda, *Targeting Immigrants.*
33. A. C. Gielen and D. Sleet, "Application of Behavior-Change Theories and Methods to Injury Prevention. *Epidemiologic Reviews* 25, no. 1 (2003): 65–76.
34. While there is a growing reliance on ecological over individual theories of health behavior, these theories also give primacy to the individual and render the environment as a unidirectional force that matters only insofar as it impacts individual health behavior. For a critique of the ecological model of health see Nancy J. Burke, et al., "Theorizing Social Context: Rethinking Behavioral Theory," *Health Education & Behavior* 36, no. 5 (2009 suppl): 55S–70S.
35. Inda, *Targeting Immigrants,* 32.
36. Nikolas Rose uses the term somatic experts. N. Rose, *The Politics of Life Itself: Biomedicine, Power and Subjectivity in the Twenty-First Century* (Princeton, NJ: Princeton University Press, 2007).
37. Rose, 33.
38. Rose, 23.
39. Inda, *Targeting Immigrants,* 38.
40. D. Lupton, *The Imperative of Health: Public Health and the Regulated Body* (Thousand Oaks, CA: Sage, 1995), 5.
41. D. Lupton, "Risk as Moral Danger: The Social and Political Functions of Risk Discourse in Public Health," *International Journal of Health Services* 23, no. 3 (1993): 425–435; Petersen and Lupton, *New Public Health*; Inda.
42. J. Bickham Mendez, "Gendered Governmentalities and Neoliberal Logics: Latina, Immigrant Women in Healthcare and Social Services," *Journal of Contemporary Ethnography* 49, no. 4 (2020): 481–506; N. Hiemstra, "Immigrant "Illegality" as Neoliberal Governmentality in Leadville, Colorado," *Antipode* 42, no. 1 (2010): 74–102.
43. N. J. Kiersey, "Everyday Neoliberalism and the Subjectivity of Crisis: Post-political Control in an Era of Financial Turmoil," *Journal of Critical Globalisation Studies*, 4 (2011): 23–44.
44. Excess death is the difference between the number of deaths observed in a racial/ethnic group and the number of deaths that would have occurred in that group if it had the same death rate as the non-Hispanic white population. For a discussion of excess death in U.S. minority populations see C. Ayala et al., "Racial/ethnic Disparities in Mortality by Stroke Subtype in the United States, 1995–1998," *American Journal of Epidemiology* 154, no. 11 (2001): 1057–1063.
45. N. K. Denzin and Y. S. Lincoln, eds., *Strategies of Qualitative Inquiry* (Thousand Oaks, CA: Sage, 2008), 2:7.

2. Structural Violence, Migrant Activism, and Indigenous Health

Epigraph: Excerpt from a speech given by Odilia Romero Hernández in April 1–4, 2012, titled "Tales from the Trenches: Developing and Defending Indigenous Identities, Rights, and Cultural Practices through Community Organizing," published by the Committee for U.S.–Latin American Relations, Cornell University, accessed August 11, 2015, http://cuslar.org/areas-of-focus/migration/odilia-romero/.

1. E. Truax, "Indígenas sin qué celebrar," *La Opinion* (digital version), August, 10, (2007).

2. E. Bermudez, "Trying out Indigenous Languages," *Los Angeles Times*, October 11, 2010.

3. S. M. Holmes, "An Ethnographic Study of the Social Context of Migrant Health in the United States," PLOS Medicine 3, no. 10 (2006): e448.

4. Holmes, "Ethnographic Study"; S. M. Holmes, "'Oaxacans Like to Work Bent Over': The Naturalization of Social Suffering among Berry Farm Workers," *International Migration* 45, no. 3 (2007): 39–68.; S. M. Holmes, *Fresh Fruit, Broken Bodies: Migrant Farmworkers in the United States* (Berkeley: University of California Press, 2013); H. Castañeda et al., "Immigration as a Social Determinant of Health," *Annual Review of Public Health*, 36 (2015): 375–392.

5. P. Farmer, *Pathologies of Power: Health, Human Rights and the New War on the Poor* (Berkeley: University of California Press 2005), 8.

6. Farmer, 8.

7. Farmer, 8–9.

8. Holmes, "Ethnographic Study."

9. C. C. Gravlee, "How Race Becomes Biology: Embodiment of Social Inequality," *American Journal of Physical Anthropology* 139, no. 1 (2009): 47–57.

10. N. Krieger, "Embodiment: A Conceptual Glossary for Epidemiology," *Journal of Epidemiology & Community Health* 59, no. 5 (2005): 350–355.

11. W. L. Duncan et al., "Lucharle por la Vida: The Impact of Migration on Health," in *Migration from the Mexican Mixteca: A Transnational Community in Oaxaca and California*, ed. Wayne A. Cornelius, David S. Fitzgerald, Jorge Hernández-Díaz, and Scott Borger (San Diego: Center for US-Mexican Studies, University of California, 2009), 165–205.

12. G. Rivera-Salgado, "From Hometown Clubs to Transnational Social Movement: The Evolution of Oaxacan Migrant Associations in California," *Social Justice* 42, no. 3/4 (142) (2015): 121.

13. J. Hubner, "Hispanic Indians: The New Workforce Almost Half of State's 330,000 Indians Have Mexican Roots—Most Are Migrants Toiling in Fields, Service Jobs," *San Jose Mercury*, August 4, 2001.

14. In addition to the devastating economic effects of free trade on corn production in the region, the introduction of genetically modified corn from the United States is having devastating environmental effects. See C. H. Cummings, "Risking Corn, Risking Culture," *World Watch* 16, no. 6 (November/December 2002).

15. D. Bacon, "NAFTA, the Cross-Border Disaster," *American Prospect*, November 7, 2017.

16. G. Otero, "Neoliberal Globalization, NAFTA, and Migration: Mexico's Loss of Food and Labor Sovereignty," *Journal of Poverty* 15, no. 4 (2011): 384–402, doi: 10.1080/10875549.2011.614514.

17. D. Harvey, *Neoliberalism: A Brief History* (Oxford: Oxford University Press, 2005), 101–102.

18. Rivera-Salgado, "From Hometown Clubs," 121.

19. J. Hubner, "Hispanic Indians: The New Workforce Almost Half of State's 330,000 Indians Have Mexican Roots—Most Are Migrants Toiling in Fields, Service Jobs," *San Jose Mercury*, August 4, 2001.

20. Jonathan Fox and Gaspar Rivera-Salgado, eds., *Indigenous Mexican Migrants in the United States* (La Jolla, CA: Center for U.S.–Mexico Studies and Center for Comparative Immigration Studies, UCSD, 2004).

21. CMACNoticias (Comunicación e Información de la Mujer Disponible para Periodistas y Medios de Comunicación Impresos y Electrónicos), translation mine, accessed August 21, 2007, http://www.cimacnoticias.com/noticias/04may/04052609.html.

22. P. Ruiz Nápoles, "Neoliberal Reforms and NAFTA in Mexico," *Economía UNAM* 14, no. 41, (May–August 2017): 75–89.

23. J. Nevins, "How High Must Operation Gatekeeper's Death Count Go?" *Los Angeles Times*, November 19, 2000.

24. Cited in J. Nevins and A. Nevins, *Operation Gatekeeper: The Rise of the "Illegal Alien" and the Making of the US-Mexico Boundary* (Hove, UK: Psychology Press, 2002), 115.

25. B. O. Hing, "The Racism and Immorality of the Operation Gatekeeper Death Trap," Border Criminologies (blog), April 13, 2015, http://bordercriminologies.law.ox.ac.uk /operation-gatekeeper-death-trap/.

26. International Organization for Migration, "Migrant Deaths Remain High Despite Sharp Fall in US–Mexico Border Crossings in 2017," February 16, 2018, https://www.iom.int /news/migrant-deaths-remain-high-despite-sharp-fall-us-mexico-border-crossings -2017.

27. S. Gilbert, "2020 Was Deadliest Year for Migrants Crossing Unlawfully into US via Arizona," *The Guardian*, January 30, 2021.

28. G. Joseph, "Why Do Border Deaths Persist When the Number of Border Crossings Is Falling?" *Propublica*, September 21, 2017, https://www.propublica.org/article /why-do-border-deaths-persist-when-the-number-of-border-crossings-is-falling.

29. Farmer, *Pathologies of Power*, 8.

30. Harvey, *Neoliberalism*, 101.

31. Harvey, 101.

32. D. Cheslow, "In Mexico a Mayor Is Killed within Hours of Taking Office," National Public Radio, January 2, 2019, https://www.npr.org/2019/01/02/681536831/in -mexico-a-mayor-is-murdered-within-hours-of-taking-office.

33. V. Newdick, "The Indigenous Woman as Victim of Her Culture in Neoliberal Mexico," *Cultural Dynamics* 17, no. 1 (2005): 89.

34. Newdick.

35. Farmer, *Pathologies of Power*, 48.

36. D. Bacon, "Can the Triquis Go Home?" *Beacon Broadside* (blog), January 24, 2012, https://www.beaconbroadside.com/broadside/2012/01/can-the-triquis-go-home -.html.

37. Bacon.

38. A. Alastair Baverstock, "Violence, Drugs Dash Mexico Triqui People's Dream of New Start Far from Home." Reuters, December 1, 2015, https://www.reuters.com/article /cnews-us-mexico-triqui-settlement-idCAKBN0TK5M920151201.

39. Braverstock.

40. D. Paris Pombo, "Promoción de Salud o Control de Nuestros Cuerpos" (paper presented at the Mexican Association of Rural Studies, October 22–26, 2007, Veracruz, Mexico). This paper was written as part of a binational collaborative project on health promotion in indigenous communities between Dolores Paris Pombo, Patricia Zavella, and Rebecca Hester; Prisca Martínez and Sandra Luz Cortés provided research assistance.

41. P. M. Martin and N. Carvajal, "Feminicide as 'Act' and 'Process': A Geography of Gendered Violence in Oaxaca," *Gender, Place & Culture* 23, no. 7 (2016): 989–1002; Telesur, "Mexico Vows to End Violence against Indigenous Women" Telesur English,

March 8, 2020, https://www.telesurenglish.net/news/Mexico-Vows-to-End-Violence-Against-Indigenous-Women-20200308-0002.html.

42. L. Velasco Ortiz, "Organizational Experiences and Female Participation among Indigenous Oaxaqueños in Baja California," in *Indigenous Mexican Migrants in the United States*, ed. Jonathan Fox and Gaspar Rivera-Salgado (La Jolla, CA: Center for U.S.–Mexico Studies and Center for Comparative Immigration Studies, UCSD, 2004), 101–124.

43. S. Falcón, "Rape as a Weapon of War: Militarized Rape at the U.S.–Mexico Border," in *Women and Migration in the U.S.-Mexico Borderlands, a Reader*, ed. Denise Segura and Patricia Zavella (Durham, NC: Duke University Press, 2007), 203–223.

44. Falcón, 203–223.

45. Falcón, 203–223.

46. Falcón, 204.

47. M. Fernandez, "You Have to Pay with Your Body: The Hidden Violence of Sexual Violence at the Border," *New York Times*, March 3, 2019.

48. J. Fox, "Indigenous Mexican Migrant Civil Society" (paper presented at LASA, Las Vegas, Nevada, October 6–9, 2004).

49. Cultural Survival, *Observations on the State of Indigenous Women's Rights in Mexico: Alternative Report Submission*," report prepared for the 70th session of the Committee on the Elimination of Discrimination against Women, Cambridge, Massachusetts, June, 2018, https://www.culturalsurvival.org/sites/default/files/CEDAW_Report_Mexico_2018.pdf.

50. See, for example, former President Trump's comments about migrants as criminals and rapists reported in "Drug Dealers, Criminals, Rapists: What Trump Thinks of Mexicans," *BBC News*, August 31, 2016, https://www.bbc.com/news/av/world-us-canada-37230916.

51. L. M. Cacho, *Social Death: Racialized Rightlessness and the Criminalization of the Unprotected* (New York: NYU Press, 2012), 4.

52. Cacho, 6.

53. L. Stephen, *Transborder Lives: Indigenous Oaxacans in Mexico, California, and Oregon*. (Durham, NC: Duke University Press, 2007), 143.

54. W. Duncan et al., "Lucharle por la Vida: The Impact of Migration on Health," in *Migration from the Mexican Mixteca: A Transnational Community in Oaxaca and California, San Diego, Estados Unidos*, ed. Wayne A. Cornelius, David Fitzgerald, Jorge Hernández-Díaz, and Scott Borger (Boulder, CO: Lynne Rienner, 2009), 193–194.

55. Holmes, "'Oaxacans Like to Work Bent Over.'"

56. L. R. Chavez, *Covering Immigration: Popular Images and the Politics of the Nation* (Berkeley: University of California Press, 2001), 176–192.

57. Holmes, "'Oaxacans Like to Work Bent Over.'"

58. Cited in Bacon, "Can the Triquis Go Home?"

59. Xochitl Castañeda discussed this in her presentation at the Summer Institute on Migration and Health in Puebla, Mexico, July 2007.

60. Office of Disease Prevention and Health Promotion, "Social Determinants of Health," http://www.healthypeople.gov/2020/topics-objectives/topic/social-determinants-health.

61. M. G. Marmot et al., "Health Inequalities among British Civil Servants: The Whitehall II Study," *Lancet* 337, no. 8754 (1991): 1387–1393.

62. M. Everett and J. N. Wieland, "Diabetes among Oaxaca's Transnational Population: An Emerging Syndemic," *Annals of Anthropological Practice* 36, no. 2 (2012): 295–311.

63. S. S. Willen et al., "Syndemic Vulnerability and the Right to Health," *Lancet* 389, no. 10072 (2017): 964–977.

64. S. Merill and S. Clair, "Syndemics and Public Health: Reconceptualizing Disease in Bio-social Context," *Medical Anthropology Quarterly* 17, no. 4 (2003): 428.

65. Everett and Wieland, "Diabetes among Oaxaca's Transnational Population."

66. Fox and Rivera-Salgado, *Indigenous Mexican Migrants*, 4.

67. B. D. Smedley et al., eds., *Unequal Treatment: Confronting Racial and Ethnic Disparities in Health Care* (Washington, DC: National Academies Press, 2002), 5.

68. Smedley et al., 6.

69. Smedley et al., 6.

70. Holmes, "An Ethnographic Study."

71. For a discussion of "driving while Triqui," see P. Johnston, "The Blossoming of Transnational Citizenship: A California Town Defends Indigenous Immigrants," in Fox and Rivera-Salgado, *Indigenous Mexican Migrants*, 385–400. Indigenous Mexicans are often exploited because they do not speak fluent Spanish and because many of them will not protest their mistreatment by employers, labor contractors, landlords, or other authority figures.

72. P. Esquivel, "Epithet That Divides Mexicans Is Banned by Oxnard School District," *LA Times*, May 28, 2012, https://www.latimes.com/local/la-xpm-2012-may-28-la-me-indigenous-derogatory-20120528-story.html.

73. V. Mendoza, "Interpretación indígena facilita la atención médica," *Californian*, June 14, 2014, https://www.thecalifornian.com/story/news/local/el-sol/2014/06/14/interpretacin-indgena-facilita-la-atencin-mdica/10496477/.

74. G. Wozniacka, "Latino-Indigenous Mexican Divide Stirs California Town," *CNSNews*, August 13, 2011, http://cnsnews.com/news/article/latino-indigenous-mexican-divide-stirs-calif-town.

75. G. Wozniacka, "Town at War: Older Immigrants vs. Newer Ones," *NBC News*, August 15, 2011, http://www.nbcnews.com/id/44151448/ns/us_news-life/t/town-war-older-immigrants-vs-newer-ones/#.XjHQq2hKg2w.

76. F. Lopez and D. Runsten, "Mixtecs and Zapotecs Working in California: Rural and Urban Experiences" (second draft of a paper presented at the conference Indígenas Mexicanos Migrantes en Estados Unidos: Construyendo Puentes entre Investigadores y Líderes Comunitarios, University of California, Santa Cruz, October 11–12, 2002).

77. D. Bacon, *Communities without Borders: Images and Voices from the World of Migration* (Ithaca, NY: ILR Press, 2006).

78. D. Bacon, "Cultivating a Community," *Contexts* 3, no. 4 (Fall 2004): 52.

79. R. Mines et al., *California's Indigenous Farmworkers*, final report of the Indigenous Farmworker Study (IFS) to the California Endowment, 2010, http://indigenousfarmworkers.org.

80. Mines et al.

81. C. Hanley, "Trailer Park's Children Played for Years on Superfund Site," *Los Angeles Times*, March 19, 2000.

82. Hanley.

83. V. R. Newkirk II, "Trump's EPA Concludes Environmental Racism Is Real," *Atlantic*, February 28, 2018.

84. L. M. Frazier, "Reproductive Disorders Associated with Pesticide Exposure," *Journal of Agromedicine* 12, no. 1 (2007): 27–37.

85. The exception to this are the Zapotecs, a predominantly urban population working in the service sector. See F. H. López and D. Runsten, "Mixtecs and Zapotecs Working in

California: Rural and Urban Experiences," in *Indigenous Mexican Migrants*, ed. Jonathan Fox and Gaspar Rivera-Salgado (La Jolla, CA: Center for U.S.-Mexico Studies and Center for Comparative Immigration Studies, UCSD, 2004), 249–278.

86. F. Fernandes, "Hunger for Jobs Forces Laborers to Put Their Health on the Line," *UC Mexus News*, 42 (Summer 2005): 7.

87. Central Coast Environmental Health Project (CCEHP), "Portrait of a Laborer: Indigenous Farmworkers in Santa Barbara County," Summer 2006.

88. B. Bade, "Sweatbaths, Sacrifice, and Surgery: The Practice of Transmedical Health Care by Mixtec Migrant Families in California" (PhD diss., University of California Riverside, 1994), https://www.proquest.com/docview/304094501?pq-origsite =gscholar&fromopenview=true.

89. B. Bade presentation at the Día del Indígena in Salinas, California, October 10, 2008.

90. L. Kresge, "Indigenous Oaxacan Communities in California: An Overview," California Institute for Rural Studies, 2007, http://lib.ncfh.org/pdfs/7340.pdf.

91. K. Moos, *Documenting Vulnerability: Food Insecurity among Indigenous Mexican Migrants in California's Central Valley* (Washington, DC: Congressional Hunger Center, 2008).

92. Holmes, An Ethnographic Study; Holmes, *Fresh Fruit, Broken Bodies*; Everett and Wieland, "Diabetes among Oaxaca's Transnational Population."

93. Holmes, "'We Come Here to Give Away Our Strength': Embodied Social Suffering, Normalization and Medical Care among Triqui Mexican Migrant Laborers" (PhD diss., University of California, San Francisco and University of California, Berkeley, 2006).

94. Farmer, *Pathologies of Power*. The term "social suffering" comes from A. Kleinman, V. Das, and M. M. Lock, eds., *Social Suffering* (Berkeley: University of California Press, 1997). The term "legal violence" comes from C. Menjívar and L. Abrego, "Legal Violence: Immigration Law and the Lives of Central American Immigrants," *American Journal of Sociology* 117, no. 5 (2012): 1380–1421.

95. Gaspar Rivera-Salgado, "Welcome to Oaxacalifornia," *Cultural Survival Quarterly Magazine*, March 1999, https://www.culturalsurvival.org/publications/cultural-survi val-quarterly/welcome-oaxacalifornia.

96. Excerpt from a speech given by Odilia Romero Hernández in April 2012 titled "Tales from the Trenches: Developing and Defending Indigenous Identities, Rights, and Cultural Practices through Community Organizing," Committee for U.S.–Latin American Relations, Cornell University, April 2012, http://cuslar.org/areas-of-focus/migration /odilia-romero/.

97. For descriptions of this activism see Fox and Rivera-Salgado, *Indigenous Mexican Migrants*.

98. See, for example, the Tequio Youth program in Oxnard, California, http://Mixtec.org /tequio. See also Oaxacalifornia Reporting Team / Equipo do Cronistas Oaxacalifornianos, Juan Santiago, *Voices of Indigenous Oaxacan Youth in the Central Valley*, Research Report No. 1, (Santa Cruz: U.C. Center for Collaborative Research for an Equitable California, UCSC, 2013).

99. C. Maldonado and P. A. Rodríguez, "'Now We Are Awake': Women's Political Participation in the Oaxacan Indigenous Binational Front," in *Indigenous Mexican Migrants*, ed. Fox and Rivera-Salgado (La Jolla, CA: Center for U.S.–Mexico Studies and Center for Comparative Immigration Studies, UCSD, 2004), 495–510; M. Blackwell, "Líderes Campesinas: Nepantla Strategies and Grassroots Organizing at the Intersection of Gender and Globalization," *Aztlán: A Journal of Chicano Studies* 35,

no. 1 (2010): 13–47; M. Blackwell, *Líderes Campesinas: Grassroots Gendered Leadership, Community Organizing, and Pedagogies of Empowerment*, prepared for NYU/Wagner Research Center for Leadership in Action, Leadership for a Changing World Research and Documentation Component, 2006, https://wagner.nyu.edu /files/leadership/Lideres.pdf.

100. S. J. Ramírez Romero, "Identidad política y derechos de los pueblos indígenas: La reconstrucción de la identidad política del Frente Indígena Oaxaqueño Binacional" (Mexico City: Comisión Nacional para el Desarrollo de los Pueblos Indígenas, 2003), 52.

101. Ramírez Romero, "Identidad política."

102. S. Escárcega and S. Varese, *La ruta mixteca* (Mexico City: Universidad Nacional Autónoma de México, 2004).

103. See Ramírez Romero, "Identidad política," for more information on the historical precursors to binational indigenous activism in Mexico and the United States.

104. P. Toy, D. Werner, and P. Stoddard, *Trainer's Guide and Toolkit* (Los Angeles: UCLA Center for Health Policy Research, Health DATA Program, Data & Democracy Train-the-Trainer Course, January 2006), https://healthpolicy.ucla.edu/programs/health -data/trainings/Documents/trainersguideandtoolkit.pdf.

105. "Oaxacan Culture: Culture Competence Guidebook," 2007, unpublished.

106. See, for example, the work of Rishi Manchanda and his organization HealthBegins in Los Angeles or the Structural Competency Working Group at UC Berkeley for examples of ways that upstream factors are screened for and assessed for their influence on health outcomes.

107. "Oaxacan Culture: Culture Competence Guidebook," 2007, unpublished.

3. The "Mexican Model" of Health

Epigraph: T. Macdonald, *Health Promotion* (London: Routledge, 1998), 28.

1. I recognize that while she may not have a car, if she is offered a ride from a friend who has a car, she will need a car seat for her child. Nonetheless, what is important for me in her reaction is that she did not perceive the information as being relevant to her life in that moment.

2. B. Bade, "Alive and Well: Generating Alternatives to Biomedical Health Care by Mixtec Migrant Families in California," in *Indigenous Mexican Migrants in the United States*, ed. Jonathan Fox and Gaspar Rivera-Salgado (La Jolla, CA: Center for U.S.-Mexican Studies and Center for Comparative Immigration Studies, UCSD, 2004), 206.

3. L. Luccisano, "The Mexican *Oportunidades* Program: Questioning the Linking of Security to Conditional Social Investments for Mothers and Children," *Canadian Journal of Latin American and Caribbean Studies* 31, no. 62 (2006): 53–85; L. Luccisano, "Mexico's Progresa Program (1997–2000): An Example of Neo-liberal Poverty Alleviation Programs Concerned with Gender, Human Capital Development, Responsibility and Choice," *Journal of Poverty* 8, no. 4 (2004): 31–57.

4. E. Kohl-Arenas, *The Self-Help Myth: How Philanthropy Fails to Alleviate Poverty*, vol. 1. (Berkeley: University of California Press, 2015), 1:25.

5. World Health Organization, *Ottawa Charter for Health Promotion*, WHO, 1986, http://www.who.int/healthpromotion/conferences/previous/ottawa/en/.

6. E. Fosse and A. Roeiseland, "From Vision to Reality? The Ottawa-Charter in Norwegian Health Policy," *Internet Journal of Health Promotion* 1 (1999).

7. World Health Organization, *Ottawa Charter*.

8. I. Kickbusch, "Models for Population Health: The Contribution of the World Health Organization to a New Public Health and Health Promotion," *American Journal of Public Health* 93, no. 3 (2003): 383–388.

9. World Health Organization, *Ottawa Charter.*

10. World Health Organization, Declaration of Alma Ata, International Conference on Primary Health Care, Alma Ata, USSR, September 6–12, 1978, https://www.who.int /publications/almaata_declaration_en.pdf.

11. J. J. Hall and R. Taylor, "Health for All beyond 2000: The Demise of the Alma Ata Declaration and Primary Health Care in Developing Countries," *Medical Journal of Australia*, 178, no.1 (January 2003):18.

12. M. Cueto, "The Origins of Primary Health Care and Selective Primary Health Care," *American Journal of Public Health* 94, no. 11 (November 2004): 1864–1874.

13. Quoted in L. A. Kaprio, "Foreword" in *Primary Health Care 2000*, ed. J. Fry and J. C. Hasler, (New York: Churchill Livingstone, 1986), vi.

14. Kaprio, "Foreword," vi–vii.

15. World Health Organization, Declaration of Alma Ata, International Conference on Primary Health Care, Alma Ata, USSR, September 6–12, 1978, https://www.who.int /publications/almaata_declaration_en.pdf.

16. See L. Chen, J. Leaning, and V. Narasimhan, "Global Health Challenges for Human Security," Global Equity Initiative, Asia Center, Harvard University, 2003. Distributed by Harvard University Press for a series of important essays on the connection between global health and human security.

17. M. Lalonde, *A New Perspective on the Health of Canadians* (Ottawa, ON: Minister of Supply and Services Canada, 1974), 5, http://www.phac-aspc.gc.ca/ph-sp/pdf /perspect-eng.pdf.

18. Lalonde, 5.

19. S. Bell, "The Development of Modern Health Promotion," in *The Social Significance of Health Promotion*, ed. Théodore MacDonald (London: Routledge, 2003), 23.

20. Lalonde, *A New Perspective*, 6.

21. Lalonde, 6.

22. Lalonde, 6.

23. J. A. Califano, "Secretary's Foreword," in *Healthy People: The Surgeon General's Report on Health Promotion and Disease Prevention* (Washington, DC: US Department of Health, Education, and Welfare, 1979), vii–x.

24. M. A. Stoto et al., eds., *Healthy People 2000: Citizens Chart the Course* (Washington, DC: Institute of Medicine, 1990), xiii.

25. David Werner, "Who Killed Primary Health Care: How the Ideal of 'Health For All' was Turned into the Reality of Worsening Health for the World's Poor," in *The New Internationalist*, HealthWrights, 1995, https://newint.org/features/1995/10/05/who.

26. World Health Organization, *Declaration of Alma Ata.* My emphasis.

27. Hall and Taylor, "Health for All," 18.

28. Cueto, "The Origins of Primary Health Care."

29. World Health Organization, *The Declaration of Alma Ata.*

30. Hall and Taylor, "Health for All," 17.

31. Cueto, "The Origins of Primary Health Care."

32. V. Valentine, "Health for the Masses: China's Barefoot Doctors," November 4, 2005, http://www.npr.org/templates/story/story.php?storyId=4990242. See also K. Dennis et al., "Community Health Workers and Promotores in California," The Center for

the Health Professions, University of California San Francisco. September 2004; For discussions of the Chinese roots of the community health workers model see E. L. Rosenthal et al., "A Summary of the National Community Health Study: Weaving the Future," a Policy Research Project of the University of Arizona, 1998.

33. V. W. Sidel and R. Sidel, "Medicine in China: Individual and Society," *Hastings Center Study* 2, no. 3 (September 1974): 24.

34. Sidel and Sidel, 24.

35. Cueto, "The Origins of Primary Health Care."

36. D. Keane, C. Nielsen, and C. Dower, *Community Health Workers and Promotores in California*, California Workforce Initiative, Community Health Workers Central (CHWC), 2004, 2, https://chwcentral.org/resources/community-health-workers-and -promotores-in-california%E2%80%8B/. Although the Chinese model was empha- sized, China did not attend the Alma Ata conference because of tensions with the USSR and because they felt they would have little to learn there. See Cueto, "The Origins of Primary Health Care." It should also be mentioned that in the United States, Native Americans were also using village health workers in the 1970s.

37. Cueto, "The Origins of Primary Health Care."

38. Cueto.

39. Cueto.

40. Cueto.

41. Cueto.

42. Cueto.

43. Cueto.

44. V. Navarro, "The World Situation and Who," *Lancet* 363, no. 9417 (April 17, 2004): 1322.

45. Hall and Taylor, "Health for All," 18.

46. C. Thomas and M. Weber, "The Politics of Global Governance: Whatever Happened to Health for All by the Year 2000?" *Global Governance* 10, no. 2 (August 2004): 187–205.

47. Italics are mine.

48. D. Lupton, *The Imperative of Health: Public Health and the Regulated Body* (Thou- sand Oaks, CA: Sage, 1995); Jonathan Xavier Inda, *Targeting Immigrants: Govern- ment, Technology, and Ethics* (Hoboken, NJ: John Wiley & Sons, 2008).

49. The term "regime of truth" comes from the writings of Michel Foucault. See M. Fou- cault, *Power/Knowledge: Selected Interviews and Other writings, 1972–1977* (New York: Pantheon Books, 1972).

50. N. Rose, "Governing 'Advanced' Liberal Democracies," in *Foucault and Political Rea- son: Liberalism, Neo-liberalism, and Rationalities of Government*, ed. Andrew Barry, Thomas Osborne, and Nikolas Rose (Chicago: University of Chicago Press, 1996), 50.

51. The term "regime of representation" comes from A. Escobar, *Encountering Develop- ment: The Making and Unmaking of the Third World* (Princeton, NJ: Princeton Uni- versity Press, 1995).

52. See Escobar for a discussion of the development apparatus.

53. K. R. Stebbins, "Politics, Economics and Health Services in Rural Oaxaca, Mexico," *Human Organization* 45, no. 2 (Summer 1986): 112–119.

54. Stebbins.

55. Rose, "Governing," 48.

56. Rose, 48.

57. L. Mills, "Maternal Health Policy and the Politics of Scale in Mexico," *Social Politics: International Studies in Gender, State and Society* 13, no. 4 (2006): 487–521.

58. A. C. Laurell, "Structural Adjustment and the Globalization of Social Policy in Latin America," *International Sociology* 15, no. 2 (2000): 315. See also A. Kleinman and J. Kleinman (1997) "The Appeal of Experience; The Dismay of Images: Cultural Appropriations of Suffering in Our Times," in *Social Suffering*, ed. A. Kleinman, V. Das, and M. Lock (Berkeley: University of California Press, 2000), for a critique of the use of DALYs as a measure of the cost of suffering from illnesses globally.

59. Laurell, "Structural Adjustment," 316.

60. B. Rasmussen-Cruz et al., "La Participación Comunitaria en Salud en el Instituto Mexican del Seguro Social en Jalisco," *Salud Pública Méx* 35, no. 5 (1993): 471–476.

61. Cited in L. Lucissano, "The Mexican *Oportunidades* Program: Questioning the Linking of Security to Conditional Social Investments for Mothers and Children," *Canadian Journal of Latin American and Caribbean Studies* 31, no. 62 (2006): 53–85. See also L. Luccisano, "Mexico's Progresa Program (1997–2000): An Example of Neoliberal Poverty Alleviation Programs Concerned with Gender, Human Capital Development, Responsibility and Choice," *Journal of Poverty* 8, no. 4 (2004): 31–57.

62. Lucissano, "The Mexican *Oportunidades* Program."

63. Lucissano, "The Mexican *Oportunidades* Program."

64. In Santiago Juxtlahuaca, Oaxaca, the doctors have a detailed map of all the health conditions observed within their regions, which they track using colored pins.

65. Lucissano, "The Mexican *Oportunidades* Program."

66. Lucissano, The Mexican *Oportunidades* Program."

67. Rose, "Governing," 49.

68. Rose, 55.

69. E. Yörük, İ. Öker, and L. Şarlak, "Indigenous Unrest and the Contentious Politics of Social Assistance in Mexico," *World Development*, 123 (2019): 104618.

70. Mills, "Maternal Health," 501. During my time in Oaxaca I heard from a number of families about what they felt was the arbitrary nature of the decision making for which family or community received Oportunidades and which did not.

71. L. Lucissano, 2002) "Mexican Anti-Poverty Programs and the Making of "Responsible" Poor Citizens (1995–2000)" (PhD diss., Department of Sociology, York University, Toronto, 2019).

72. J. Ferguson, *Give a Man a Fish: Reflections on the New Politics of Distribution* (Durham, NC: Duke University Press, 2015).

73. McGregor, S. "Neoliberalism and Health Care," *International Journal of Consumer Studies*, 25, no. 2 (June 2001): 82–89.

74. Inda, *Targeting Immigrants*, 13.

75. Trade-Related Intellectual Property Rights (TRIPS) upholds and regulates a property rights system in which pharmaceutical companies who own the intellectual property rights to the drugs they make (even when the ingredients come from natural and sources) can charge whatever they like for those drugs to "developing" countries whose populations are in need of cheap drugs for chronic and life-threatening conditions, such as HIV. TRIPS is, therefore, a key player in enclosing what have been referred to as the "global commons" and stands in the way of governments and populations being able to ensure people's human right to health care. See Peter Drahos and John Braithwaite, *Information Feudalism: Who Owns the Knowledge Economy?* (London: Earthscan, 2002).

76. Hall and Taylor, "Health for All," 18.

77. Fosse and Roeiseland, "From Vision."

78. Thomas and Weber, "The Politics," 3.

79. Although this was the conception, the on-the-ground practice was not always in line with the theory, even in the early years.

80. I. Kickbusch, Keynote address, *Healthy People Consortium Meeting 2000*, November 1996, http://odphp.osophs.dhhs.gov/pubs/HP2000/kickbusch.htm.

81. J. Ferguson, "The Anti-Politics Machine," in *The Anthropology of Politics: A Reader in Ethnography, Theory and Critique*, ed. Joan Vincent (Malden, MA: Blackwell Publishing, 2002), 406.

82. I. Kickbusch and D. Gleicher, *Governance for Health in the 21st Century* (Geneva: World Health Organization, 2012).

83. Laurell, "Structural Adjustment," 316.

4. Números, Números, Números

Epigraph: Quote attributed to sociologist William Bruce Cameron.

1. R. S. Safeer and J. Kennan, "Health Literacy: The Gap between Physicians and Patients," *American Family Physician* 72, no. 3 (2005): 463–468.

2. R. Mines et al., *California's Indigenous Farmworkers*, final report of the Indigenous Farmworker Study (IFS) to the California Endowment, 2010, http://indigenousfarm workers.org.

3. M. Power, *The Audit Society: Rituals of Verification* (Oxford: Oxford University Press, 1997).

4. C. Shore and S. Wright, "Governing by Numbers: Audit Culture, Rankings and the New World Order" *Social Anthropology* 23, no. 1 (2015): 22–28.

5. C. Shore and S. Wright, , "Audit Culture Revisited: Rankings, Ratings, and the Reassembling of Society" *Current Anthropology* 56, no. 3 (2015): 431–432.

6. T. M. Porter, *Trust in Numbers: The Pursuit of Objectivity in Science and Public Life* (Princeton: Princeton University Press, 1996).

7. Porter, ix.

8. M. Strathern, *Audit Cultures: Anthropological Studies in Accountability, Ethics, and the Academy* (London: Routledge, 2000).

9. Shore and Wright,. "Audit Culture Revisited."

10. K. Mercado Asencio, "The Under-Registration of Births in Mexico: Consequences for Children, Adults, and Migrants," Migration Policy Institute, April 12, 2012, https:// www.migrationpolicy.org/article/under-registration-births-mexico-consequences -children-adults-and-migrants.

11. L. Stephen, *Transborder Lives: Indigenous Oaxacans in Mexico, California, and Oregon* (Durham, NC: Duke University Press, 2007), 143.

12. L. Silverman, "'Living, Breathing Archaeology' in the Arizona Desert," NPR, *All Things Considered*, March 24, 2012, https://www.npr.org/2012/03/24/149171195 /living-breathing-archeology-in-the-arizona-desert.

13. Maria Hotchkiss and Jessica Phelan, "Uses of Census Bureau Data in Federal Funds Distribution," U.S. Census Bureau, September 2017, https://www.census.gov/library /working-papers/2017/decennial/census-data-federal-funds.html.

14. L. Gutierrez Nájera, "Beyond National Origins: Latin@ American Indigenous Migration," *American Anthropologist* 116, no.1 (2014): 8.

15. E. Dyson, "The Quantification of Everything," Huffington Post, May 25, 2011, https:// www.huffingtonpost.com/esther-dyson/the-quantification-of-eve_b_127288.html.

16. R. Domínguez Santos, "The FIOB Experience: Internal Crisis and Future Challenges" in *Indigenous Mexican Migrants in the United States*, ed. Jonathan Fox and Gaspar Rivera-Salgado (La Jolla: University of California San Diego, Center for U.S.–Mexico Studies and Center for Comparative Immigration Studies, 2004), 69–79.

17. D. Sontag, "Immigrants Facing Deportation by US Hospitals," *New York Times*, August 3, 2008.

18. M. L. Berk and C. L. Schur, "The Effect of Fear on Access to Care among Undocumented Latino Immigrants," *Journal of Immigrant Health* 3, no. 3 (2001): 151–156; A. N. Ortega, et al., "Health Care Access, Use of Services, and Experiences among Undocumented Mexicans and Other Latinos," *Archives of Internal Medicine* 167, no. 21 (2007): 2354–2360; K. P. Derose, J. J. Escarce, and N. Lurie, "Immigrants and Health Care: Sources of Vulnerability," *Health Affairs* 26, no. 5 (2007): 1258–1268.

19. See B. Bade, "Sweatbaths, Sacrifice, and Surgery: The Practice of Transmedical Health Care by Mixtec Migrant Families in California" (PhD diss., University of California, Riverside, 1994); D. Villarejo, et al., *Suffering in Silence: A Report on the Health of California's Farmworkers* (Davis: California Institute for Rural Studies, 2000); E. Cardenas, *Portrait of a Laborer: Indigenous Farmworkers in Santa Barbara County* (Santa Barbara, CA: Central Coast Environmental Health Project, 2006); L. Kresge, *Indigenous Oaxacan Communities in California: An Overview* (Davis: California Institute for Rural Studies, 2007).

20. M. S. Danielson and T. A. Eisenstadt, "Walking Together, but in Which Direction? Gender Discrimination and Multicultural Practices in Oaxaca, Mexico," *Politics and Gender* 5, no. 2 (2009): 153–184.

21. A. Giddens, *Modernity and Self-Identity: Self and Society in the Late Modern Age* (Stanford, CA: Stanford University Press, 1991), cited in Alan Petersen, "Risk and the Regulated Self: The Discourse of Health Promotion as Politics of Uncertainty," *Australian and New Zealand Journal of Sociology* 32, no. 1 (1996): 46.

22. For a description of preventive measures used by the Triqui from San Juan Copala, Oaxaca, to care for their children see Zuanilda Mendoza González, "¿ Enfermedad para quién?: Saber popular entre los triquis" *Nueva Antropología* 16, no. 53 (1997): 117–139.

23. U. Beck, *Risk Society: Towards a New Modernity* (London: Sage, 1992).

24. Shore and Wright., "Audit Culture Revisited," 423.

25. Shore and Wright, 42.

26. M. Strathern, "The Tyranny of Transparency," *British Educational Research Journal* 26, no.3 (2000): 309–321.

5. Cultural Sensitivity Training and the Cultural Politics of Teaching Tolerance

Epigraph: M. Kearney, "Mixtec Political Consciousness: From Passive to Active Resistance," in *Rural Revolt in Mexico: US Intervention and the Domain of Subaltern Politics*, ed. Daniel Nugent, Gilbert M. Joseph, and Emily S. Rosenberg (Durham, NC: Duke University Press, 1998), 137.

1. J. Foley, "New Sex Charges in 'Marriage' Case," *Californian*, January, 14, 2009, www.thecalifornian.com.

2. Although this is what the police found out, the girl claimed to have been kidnapped when the matter went to court. V. Hennessey, "Greenfield Girl Testifies She was Kidnapped by Teen," *Monterey Herald*, January 31, 2009.

3. For a discussion of Triqui wedding practices see U. López García, "Sa'vi: Discursos Ceremoniales de Yutsa To'on (Apoala)" (PhD diss., Leiden University, 2007). It is important to note that although the legal age for marriage in California is eighteen, teenagers under eighteen are allowed to get married with parental consent, a fact that was not discussed in the media reports. In other words, underage marriage is not just a phenomenon that happens in the Triqui culture but is a common enough occurrence in California to have some laws codified regarding the practice.

4. L. Parsons, "Alleged Marriage Deal for Daughter Shows Clash of Rural Mexican, U.S. Cultures," *Mercury News*, January, 13, 2009.

5. Parsons.

6. F. Foley, "Feds Ask for Files in 'Sale' of Greenfield Girl," *Californian*, January, 14, 2009.

7. Parsons, "Alleged Marriage Deal."

8. Parsons.

9. J. Trahan, "Dad Sold 14-Year-Old Daughter to 18-Year-Old Man," *Dallas Morning News, Crime Blog*, January 14, 2009.

10. Trahan.

11. Associated Press, "Greenfield Man arrested in Teen Marriage Deal," *San Jose Mercury News*, January 13, 2009, https://www.mercurynews.com/2009/01/13/police-green field-man-arrested-in-teen-marriage-deal/.

12. L. R. Chavez, *Covering Immigration: Popular Images and the Politics of the Nation* (Berkeley: University of California Press, 2001); J. X. Inda, *Targeting Immigrants: Government, Technology, and Ethics* (Malden, MA: Blackwell, 2008).

13. S. P. Huntington, *Who Are We? The Challenges to America's National Identity* (New York: Simon and Shuster, 2004).

14. See P. Johnston, "The Blossoming of Transnational Citizenship: A California Town Defends Indigenous Immigrants," in *Indigenous Mexican Migrants in the United States*, ed. Jonathan Fox and Gaspar Rivera-Salgado (La Jolla, CA: Center for U.S.–Mexican Studies and Center for Comparative Immigration Studies, UCSD, 2004), 385–400.

15. G. Jordan G. and C. Weedon, *Cultural Politics: Class, Gender, Race and the Postmodern World* (Oxford: Blackwell, 1995), 4.

16. G. Rivera-Salgado, and R. Domínguez-Santos, "FIOB's Statement on the Case of Marcelino De Jesus Martinez," *El Enemigo Común*, January 15, 2009; E. Stanley, "Indígenas en el Banquillo: Los Triquis de California," Hispanic LA, 2009, https://hispanicla .com/indigenas-al-banquillo-1166. The exact quote in Spanish from Seth Holmes is this: "¿Quiénes son los estadounidenses para decir que su forma de casarse es mejor que la de los Triquis, especialmente cuando el 50 por ciento de esos casamientos terminan en divorcios?"

17. Jordan and Weedon, *Cultural Politics*, 5.

18. Johnston, "The Blossoming," 385–399.

19. Johnston.

20. E. Bermudez, "Protests over Police Shooting Resonate All the Way to Guatemala," *LA Times*, September 26, 2010.

21. J. Hing, "Protests, Outrage after LAPD Kills Guatemalan Father of Three," *Colorlines*, September 9, 2010.

22. Fox and Rivera-Salgado, *Indigenous Mexican Migrants*, 23.

23. P. J. DeMuniz, "Introduction," in *Immigrants in Courts*, ed. Joanne I. Moore and Margaret E. Fisher (Seattle: University of Washington Press, 1999), 3–7, cited in Daniel J.

Procaccini, "What We Have Here Is a Failure to Communicate: An Approach for Evaluating Credibility in America's Multilingual Courtrooms," *Boston College Third World Law Journal* 31, no. 1 (2011), 162–192.

24. DeMuniz, "Introduction."

25. Fox and Rivera-Salgado, *Indigenous Mexican Migrants*, 23.

26. C. Von Quednow, "Speaking English a Requirement for Motherhood?: Reunite Cirila Baltazar Cruz with Her Baby," *Colorlines*, June 15, 2009.

27. J. Elliott Jr., "Mexican Immigrant Sues after Newborn Seized by Mississippi Agency," *Mercury News*, March 12, 2014; Southern Poverty Law Center, "Federal Court Delivers Important Victory in SPLC Case against Hospital, State Employees Accused of Taking Baby from Immigrant Mother," *SPLCNews*, March 12, 2014.

28. Jordan and Weedon, *Cultural Politics*, 5.

29. On one occasion Luz could not be present, so Yadira Lopez (a pseudonym), a Zapotec woman who was affiliated with BIRM, took her place.

30. R. E. Spector, *Cultural Diversity in Health and Illness*, 6th ed. (Needham, MA: Pearson Prentice Hall, 2004).

31. The unpaid labor that Tequio relies on is often misunderstood by outsiders to be voluntary labor when, in fact, it is obligatory. Thanks to Jonathan Fox for pointing this out.

32. La Agencia, "Oaxacan Culture: Cultural Competence Guidebook" (unpublished manuscript, 2007).

33. B. Bade, "Alive and Well: Generating Alternatives to Biomedical Health Care by Mixtec Migrant Families in California," in *Indigenous Mexican Migrants*, ed. Jonathan Fox and Gaspar Rivera-Salgado (La Jolla, CA: Center for U.S.–Mexican Studies and Center for Comparative Immigration Studies, UCSD, 2004), 205–247.

34. For more information about the education levels of indigenous Mexican migrant children see R. Mines, S. Nichols, and D. Runsten, "Final Report of the Indigenous Farmworker Study (IFS) to the California Endowment," 2010, http://indigenousfarm workers.org/index.shtml.

35. W. Mignolo, "Epistemic Disobedience: The De-colonial Option and the Meaning of Identity in Politics," *Gragoatá*, no. 22 (1st semester 2007): 26.

36. Mignolo.

37. L. Stephen, *Transborder Lives: Indigenous Oaxacans in Mexico, California, and Oregon* (Durham, NC: Duke University Press, 2007), 57.

38. This man was supposed to stay for three years, although Jeronimo, who is from the same village, doubted that he would stay that long. While three years is an exceptionally long time for him to be required to stay in the village to fulfill his cargo, this particular clinic had a doctor who demanded that "her" Comité de Salud stay in residence for three years because she did not want to train new members each year. This demand was both tragic and comic in that the man we met was only responsible for keeping the keys to the clinic, opening and closing the doors each day, a job that required very little training. While he spent his days waiting to open and close the clinic, his wife and children were in Fresno waiting for his return. The price was worth it to him, however. He revealed to us that his house, which was one of the largest in the village as far as I could tell, was almost built, and he did not want to jeopardize its construction or his standing in the community.

39. E. Papps and I. Ramsden, "Cultural Safety in Nursing: The New Zealand Experience," *International Journal for Quality in Health Care* 8, no. 5 (1996): 491–497.

40. The word for sensitive in Spanish is *sensible* (pronounced sen-see'-blay). Jeronimo's mistranslation of this false cognate amused many of the sympathetic service

providers in the room who knowingly looked at each other, nodding their heads and saying, "Yeah, we do need to be more sensible in our interactions with this population."

41. W. Brown, *Regulating Aversion: Tolerance in the Age of Identity and Empire* (Princeton, NJ: Princeton University Press, 2006), 13.
42. Brown, 14.
43. Brown, 15.
44. Brown, 16.
45. G. Pon, "Cultural Competency as New Racism: An Ontology of Forgetting," *Journal of Progressive Human Services* 20, no. 1 (2009): 60.
46. Pon, 60.
47. Mignolo, "Epistemic Disobedience," 32.
48. M. Foucault, *Power/Knowledge: Selected Interviews and Other Writings, 1972–1977* (New York: Pantheon Books, 1972), 197.
49. T. Asad, "From the History of Colonial Anthropology to the Anthropology of Western Hegemony," in *Colonial Situations: Essays on the Contextualization of Ethnographic Knowledge*, ed. George Stocking (Madison, WI: University of Wisconsin Press), 316.
50. See the work of Sylvia Wynter for a discussion of this issue.
51. Jordan and Weedon, *Cultural Politics*, 253.
52. S. Hall, "Culture, Identity and Diaspora," in *Identity: Community, Culture, Difference*, ed. Jonathan Rutherford (London: Lawrence and Wishart, 1990), 225–226.
53. J. M. Metzl and D. E. Roberts, "Structural Competency Meets Structural Racism: Race, Politics, and the Structure of Medical Knowledge," *American Medical Association Journal of Ethics* 16, no. 9 (2014): 674–690.
54. I. Sakamoto, "An Anti-oppressive Approach to Cultural Competence," *Canadian Social Work Review/Revue Canadienne de Service Social* 24, no. 1 (2007): 105–114.
55. Pon, "Cultural Competency."
56. C. Hale, "Activist Research v. Cultural Critique: Indigenous Land Rights and the Contradictions of Politically Engaged Anthropology," *Cultural Anthropology* 21, no. 1 (2006): 96–120.
57. Hale, 111.

6. La Lucha Sigue

La lucha sigue means "the struggle continues." It is a common refrain in migrant activist circles.

1. D. Lupton, *The Imperative of Health: Public Health and the Regulated Body* (Thousand Oaks, CA: Sage, 1995), 6.
2. B. Bade, "Alive and Well: Generating Alternatives to Biomedical Health Care by Mixtec Migrant Families in California," in *Indigenous Mexican Migrants*, ed. Jonathan Fox and Gaspar Rivera-Salgado (La Jolla, CA: Center for U.S.–Mexican Studies and Center for Comparative Immigration Studies, UCSD, 2004), 233.
3. J. M. Metzl, "Structural Competency," *American Quarterly* 64, no. 2 (2012): 213–218.
4. J. S. Taylor, "Confronting "Culture" in Medicine's "Culture of No Culture," *Academic Medicine* 78, no. 6 (2003): 555–559.
5. A. Dávila, *Latinos, Inc.: The Marketing and Making of a People* (Berkeley: University of California Press, 2012).
6. S. M. Holmes, *Fresh Fruit, Broken Bodies: Migrant Farmworkers in the United States*, vol. 27 (Berkeley: University of California Press, 2013), 195.

7. G. Pon, "Cultural Competency as New Racism: An Ontology of Forgetting," *Journal of Progressive Human Services* 20, no. 1 (2009): 59–71; E. A. Viruell-Fuentes, P. Y. Miranda, and S. Abdulrahim, "More Than Culture: Structural Racism, Intersectionality Theory, and Immigrant Health," *Social science & medicine* 75, no. 12 (2012): 2099–2106.

8. M. K. Singer et al., "Culture: The Missing Link in Health Research," *Social Science & Medicine*, 170 (2016): 237–246.

9. Singer et al.

10. J. S. Taylor, Confronting "Culture" in Medicine's "Culture of No Culture," *Academic Medicine*, 78, no. 6 (2003): 555–559.

11. Holmes, *Fresh Fruit*, 196.

12. K. Olcoń and L. E. Gulbas, "'Because That's the Culture': Providers' Perspectives on the Mental Health of Latino Immigrant Youth," *Qualitative Health Research* 28, no. 12 (2018): 1944–1954.

13. See, for example, the work of Vicente Navarro, Peter Waitzkin, Nancy Schepher-Hughes, Jaime Breilh, and Leo Chavez.

14. See, for example, the work of Paul Farmer, Jonathan Metzl, Helena Hansen, and Seth Holmes.

15. R. Manchanda, *The Upstream Doctors: Medical Innovators Track Sickness to Its Source* (TED Books, 2013).

16. D. Costa, "Trump Administration Looking to Cut the Already Low Wages of H-2A Migrant Farmworkers While Looking to Give Their Bosses a Multi-billion Dollar Bailout," Economic Policy Institute, April 14, 2020) https://www.epi.org/blog/trump-administration-reportedly-looking-to-cut-the-already-low-wages-of-h-2a-migrant-farmworkers-while-giving-their-bosses-a-multibillion-dollar-bailout/.

17. Costa.

18. Costa.

19. H. Bottemiller Evich, X. Bustillo, and L. Crampton, "Harvest of Shame: Farmworkers Face Coronavirus Disaster," Politico, September 8, 2020, https://www.politico.com/news/2020/09/08/farmworkers-coronavirus-disaster-409339; S. Ferris, "Hidden Hardships: Guest Farmworkers with Visas Died of COVID-19 in Obscurity While Trump Planned Wage Freezes," The Center for Public Integrity, December 23, 2020, https://publicintegrity.org/inequality-poverty-opportunity/immigration/guest-farm-workers-visas-trump-wage-freezes/; R. Jervis et al., "Worked to Death: Latino Farmworkers Have Long Been Denied Basic Rights. Covid-19 Showed How Deadly Racism Could Be," *USA Today*, October 24, 2020.

20. V. Ho, "Covid and California's Farmworkers: Study Lays Bare Disproportionate Risks," *The Guardian*, December 2, 2020.

21. Bottemiller Evich, "Harvest of Shame."

22. Bottemiller Evich.

Index

About the Author

Rebecca J. Hester is an assistant professor in the Department of Science, Technology, and Society at Virginia Tech in Blacksburg, Virginia. She is a coeditor of *Translocalities/Translocalidades: Feminist Politics of Translation in the Latin/a Américas* and the author of several publications on the promises and pitfalls of cultural competence.

Available titles in the Critical Issues in Health and Medicine series:

Laura L. Heinemann, *Transplanting Care: Shifting Commitments in Health and Care in the United States*

Rebecca J. Hester, *Embodied Politics: Indigenous Migrant Activism, Cultural Competency, and Health Promotion in California*

Laura D. Hirshbein, *American Melancholy: Constructions of Depression in the Twentieth Century*

Laura D. Hirshbein, *Smoking Privileges: Psychiatry, the Mentally Ill, and the Tobacco Industry in America*

Timothy Hoff, *Practice under Pressure: Primary Care Physicians and Their Medicine in the Twenty-first Century*

Beatrix Hoffman, Nancy Tomes, Rachel N. Grob, and Mark Schlesinger, eds., *Patients as Policy Actors*

Ruth Horowitz, *Deciding the Public Interest: Medical Licensing and Discipline*

Powel Kazanjian, *Frederick Novy and the Development of Bacteriology in American Medicine*

Claas Kirchhelle, *Pyrrhic Progress: The History of Antibiotics in Anglo-American Food Production*

Rebecca M. Kluchin, *Fit to Be Tied: Sterilization and Reproductive Rights in America, 1950–1980*

Jennifer Lisa Koslow, *Cultivating Health: Los Angeles Women and Public Health Reform*

Jennifer Lisa Koslow, *Exhibiting Health: Public Health Displays in the Progressive Era*

Susan C. Lawrence, *Privacy and the Past: Research, Law, Archives, Ethics*

Bonnie Lefkowitz, *Community Health Centers: A Movement and the People Who Made It Happen*

Ellen Leopold, *Under the Radar: Cancer and the Cold War*

Barbara L. Ley, *From Pink to Green: Disease Prevention and the Environmental Breast Cancer Movement*

Sonja Mackenzie, *Structural Intimacies: Sexual Stories in the Black AIDS Epidemic*

Stephen E. Mawdsley, *Selling Science: Polio and the Promise of Gamma Globulin*

Frank M. McClellan, *Healthcare and Human Dignity: Law Matters*

Michelle McClellan, *Lady Lushes: Gender, Alcohol, and Medicine in Modern America*

David Mechanic, *The Truth about Health Care: Why Reform Is Not Working in America*

Richard A. Meckel, *Classrooms and Clinics: Urban Schools and the Protection and Promotion of Child Health, 1870–1930*

Terry Mizrahi, *From Residency to Retirement: Physicians' Careers over a Professional Lifetime*

Manon Parry, *Broadcasting Birth Control: Mass Media and Family Planning*

Alyssa Picard, *Making the American Mouth: Dentists and Public Health in the Twentieth Century*

Heather Munro Prescott, *The Morning After: A History of Emergency Contraception in the United States*

Sarah B. Rodriguez, *The Love Surgeon: A Story of Trust, Harm, and the Limits of Medical Regulation*

David J. Rothman and David Blumenthal, eds., *Medical Professionalism in the New Information Age*

Andrew R. Ruis, *Eating to Learn, Learning to Eat: School Lunches and Nutrition Policy in the United States*

James A. Schafer Jr., *The Business of Private Medical Practice: Doctors, Specialization, and Urban Change in Philadelphia, 1900–1940*